The Pocket Review of Surgery

The
Pocket Review
of
Surgery

Sergio Huerta, M.D.
Surgical Resident (R2)
Department of Surgery
University of California, Irvine
UCI Medical Center

Theodore X. O'Connell, M.D.
Family Practice Resident (R2)
Department of Family Medicine
Santa Monica - UCLA Medical Center

J&S

J & S PUBLISHING COMPANY, INC.
ALEXANDRA, VIRGINIA

J&S

Editor: Kurt E. Johnson, Ph.D.
Printing Supervisor: Robert Perotti, Jr.
Printing: Goodway Graphics of Virginia, Inc.

Libary of Congress Catalog Card Number: 98-075657

ISBN: 1-888308-06-0

10   9   8   7   6   5   4   3   2   1

To Hsiao Ching Li, my wife, for her enormous support and help throughout the writing of every single page of this book.

Sergio Huerta, M.D.
October, 1999

To all of my teachers, who have educated and inspired me. To my parents, for being the greatest teachers of all. And to Susan, whose example drives me to be my best.

Ted O'Connell, M.D.
October, 1999

Contents

Foreword

A few years ago I was asked to teach chemistry to a group of undergraduate students who were preparing for the Medical College Admissions Test (MCAT). Since I enjoy teaching, I am usually very enthusiastic about any teaching position I can obtain. However, the situation in this case was different because my background is not in chemistry. I obtained a B.S. degree in biology from University of California, Los Angeles (UCLA) before entering medical school. Over four years had elapsed since I had studied any chemistry and I was unsure if I could do a good job teaching a subject without a strong background in the subject I was to teach.

I soon realized that not having a background in chemistry forced me to study each topic I had to present. I taught the material as I was learning it and as it made sense to me. I made no assumptions about anyone's knowledge because the material was equally hard for me. This is different from when I teach biology because I find myself not explaining concepts as well as I should. I often omit key concepts that I consider basic, incorrectly assuming that my pupils share my background. I did not encountered this in chemistry because all the concepts reviewed were new and I had to dissect them carefully to be able to explain them to others.

To my surprise, students were very pleased at the end of the five-week course. They indicated to me that among many things they were finally able to "see the big picture." They understood why they had to memorize complicated equations and quantum numbers. In addition, they had an opportunity to ask very simple questions that they never dared to ask others.

This experience made me realize that in some cases, having a strong background on a specific subject may be deleterious in teaching. This is particularly true for introductory courses; however, this is different when an individual is teaching an advanced course. When the audience has a strong background on a specific subject, a teacher who is expert on the subject material should teach it. Yet, I believe students benefit more from nonexperts when learning introductory material.

I am now just starting my second year of surgical training a fourth year medical student at the University of California, Irvine. Thus, my background in surgery is limited to my major core rotation in medical school, a few electives as a forth year medical student, and a bit over a year of surgical residency training. Therefore, I think that this book is ideal for the student who seeks information in surgery as an introductory course. I am fortunate to have had the opportunity to write this book. I hope I can succeed in introducing concepts in surgery to all those students interested in this area of medicine. Only the reader will decide if I have met my objective.

Sergio Huerta, M.D.
February, 2000

No field of medicine exists in a vacuum. We all interact with one another for clinical consults, subspecialty care, primary care, new research developments, the communication of new information, and friendship. The pediatrician may call on a surgical oncologist, a neurosurgeon may consult with a physical therapist, and the cardiothoracic surgeon may team up with an internist. Despite all of the diversification and subspecialization in medicine, we all rely on one another for the good of our patients.

It was with this philosophy in mind that I began this project. As a medical student, I often struggled to wade through the details to grasp the basic information before going back to master the details. We hope that this book will provide a solid foundation for the medical student as he or she goes through the surgery clerkship. This book is not intended to be all-encompassing. Instead, we hope that it will provide a core of important information and serve as a springboard for seeking out more detailed information. It should be used as a companion to a good surgical textbook and can be used as a helpful pocket reference to prepare for pimping during rounds.

While we are not all going to be surgeons, we will all be physicians and should thus share some common knowledge. The information contained in this book is important for budding surgeons and all other physicians alike. For it is in our patients' best interests that we know as much as possible and learn to interact with one another, not as isolated specialists, but as a team of physicians working together to help our patients.

Theodore X. O'Connell, M.D.
February, 2000

Contributing Editors

WILLIAM J. ARONSON, M.D., F.A.C.S.
Assistant Clinical Professor, Department of Urology, UCLA School of Medicine, Los Angeles

J. DENNIS BAKER, M.D.
Professor of Surgery, UCLA School of Medicine, Los Angeles
Chief of Vascular Surgery, West Los Angeles Department of Veterans Affairs Medical Center

ERIC W. FONKALSRUD, M.D.
Professor and Chief of Pediatric Surgery, UCLA School of Medicine, Los Angeles

EDWARD H. LIVINGSTON, M.D., F.A.C.S.
Director, Surgery and Perioperative Services, Veterans Administration Greater Los Angeles Healthcare System
Associate Professor of Surgery, UCLA School of Medicine, Los Angeles

THEODORE X. O'CONNELL, M.D., F.A.C.S.
Chief of Surgical Oncology, Kaiser Permanente Medical Center Los Angeles
Associate Clinical Professor of Surgical Oncology, UCLA School of Medicine, Los Angeles

MARK SAWICKI, M.D.
Assistant Professor of Surgery, Department of Surgery, Division of General Surgery, UCLA School of Medicine

MARILENE B. WANG, M.D.
Assistant Professor of Surgery, Division of Head and Neck Surgery, UCLA School of Medicine, Los Angeles
Chief of Otolaryngology, West Los Angeles Veterans Administration Medical Center

1 | GENERAL PRINCIPLES

TRAUMA

Resuscitation

- The main goal of a trauma team in the resuscitative effort is to keep the brain intact in the face of vital organ failure.
- As brain survival depends on adequate oxygenation, the aim of the resuscitation is to maintain adequate perfusion to the brain.
- In the Advanced Trauma Life Support (ATLS) protocol, the steps in resuscitation are as follows:

ATLS
1. Revival
2. Examination of vital functions
3. Definitive care

Revival

- The steps involved in revival can easily be remembered by the mnemonic A→B→C→D→E→F. The arrows indicate that these steps must be followed in a sequential order.

A= Airway
B= Breathing
C= Circulation
D= Decompression
E= Exposure
F= Fluids

Airway

- Management of the airway involves ensuring that there is a clear path for air to get into the lungs.
- Assessment should include checking for the presence of foreign objects such as dentures or blood obstructing the airway.

- In the unconscious patient, the **most common type of obstruction is the patient's own tongue** which can be quickly cleared by **chin lift and/or jaw thrust**.
- If the patient is conscious, provide evidence that airway is patent.
- Care should be taken with the patient suspected to have neck injury when establishing airway patency as neurological damage may occur. In this case the **jaw should not be elevated** and spinal immobilization should be performed.
- Neck injury should always be assumed until ruled out clinically or by x-ray.
- If a patient is tachypneic or has labored inspiration, endotracheal intubation may be needed.
- The **threshold for intubation should be low** as patients can be safely extubated on subsequent evaluation if the patient did not need endotracheal intubation.
- This is a preferred event over the need to perform an immediate intubation after the initial assessment.
- If the patient is in respiratory distress and endotracheal intubation is not successful, a cricothyroidotomy (surgical airway) should be performed.

Breathing

- Once a clear airway has been established, appropriate **breathing** should be assessed.
- Inspection of the chest as it rises should indicate air movement.
- This is followed by auscultation of the lungs for inflow/outflow of air. Lung auscultation is also needed in trauma to rule out pneumothorax.
- If the patient is not moving air, mechanical **ventilation** should be started.
- If ventilation equipment is not available, ventilation should be done by Ambu bag.
- Assessment of breathing also includes evaluation of life-threatening conditions that require prompt diagnosis such as tension/open pneumothorax, hemothorax, flail chest, and cardiac tamponade.

  - **Pneumothorax/ Hemothorax.** If either is suspected (subcutaneus emphysema, tachypnea, pleuritic pain, hypotension), a chest tube should be placed. This is best accomplished by making an incision in the fourth intercostal space above the rib and inserting of a chest tube.
  - **Flail chest** usually occurs when there are multiple rib fractures resulting in paradoxical movement of the chest with respiration. Intubation with positive pressure ventilation should be promptly started.
  - **Cardiac tamponade** occurs when there is bleeding in the pericardium resulting in impaired cardiac contractions. The diagnosis is a clinical one and consists of decreased heart sounds, jugular venous distension (JVD), and decreased blood pressure (**Beck's triad**). Immediate (IV) fluids and pericardiocentesis should be performed.

Circulation

- Circulation is quickly assessed by carotid or femoral pulse palpation.
- Presence of either of these pulses ensures a systolic blood pressure of at least 60mm Hg even in the absence of radial pulses.
- Capillary refill (< 2 seconds) and skin color are also good indicators of adequate perfusion.
- If pulses are not palpable, Cardiopulmonary Resuscitation (CPR) should be started. Chest compressions of 1.5-2.0 inches at a rate of 80-100 times/ minute should provide adequate brain perfusion.
- If the heart sounds are present, positioning the patient at -30° (Trendelenburg's position) optimizes blood flow to the brain.
- The next step consists of establishing adequate venous access, which is usually accomplished by placement of two 16-gauge or larger peripheral IV lines. While obtaining IV access, blood can be obtained to perform the following tests:

BLOOD TESTS
1. Blood sample for type and crossmatch x 6 units of blood
2. Culture
3. CBC, electrolytes, BUN, creatinine

- If marked hypotension is present, the source of shock must be investigated.
- **If shock is present in the trauma patient, the threshold to give O⁻ blood should be low.**

TYPES OF SHOCK
- **Hypovolemic shock** occurs as a result of vascular contraction due to decreased blood volume. This may be as a result of bleeding or severe dehydration. Dry mucous membranes, ↓JVD, and tachycardia are common manifestations of hypovolemic shock. Treatment should be aimed at volume repletion.
- **Cardiogenic shock** occurs as a result of failure of the heart to pump (i.e., congestive heart failure [CHF]). In contrast to hypovolemic shock, patients in cardiogenic shock have evidence of fluid overload (i.e., JVD, edema). Fluid should be administered with care in these patients. Treatment with cardiotonic drugs is the mainstay of treatment.
- **Neurogenic shock** occurs due to loss of vascular tone following spinal cord injury. Treatment is aimed at increasing the peripheral vascular resistance with vasoconstrictive drugs.
- **Septic shock** occurs as a result of endotoxin release by bacteria. Broad-spectrum antibiotics should be quickly administered to treat the infectious process. Supportive care should include vasopressors and IV fluids.

- Once **A**irway, **B**reathing and **C**irculation have been adequately attended to, a brief history should be obtained from the patient or relatives.

- The patient should be reassured and informed as to the situation and planned steps in management.

- The mnemonic **AMPLE** can be used to remember salient aspects in obtaining a quick history from the trauma patient.

    A= Allergies
    M= Medications
    P= Past medical history
    L= Last meal
    E= Events preceding the emergency

Decompression

- The trauma patient should receive gastric decompression with a nasogastric tube. This reduces the risk of aspiration in patients with emesis.

- Decompression of the bladder should also be done by placement of a Foley catheter. In addition, a Foley catheter is a reliable way to assess urine output and thus adequate hydration status. If possible, urethral injury should be ruled out before placement of a Foley catheter . A displaced prostate may be suggested by rectal examination. If this is the case a urethrogram is recommended to rule out urethral injury.

Exposure

- Complete disrobing allows a thorough examination by inspection and palpation of the trauma patient.

- The trauma patient should be kept warm to avoid hypothermia and discomfort.

Fluids

- Aggressive fluid resuscitation should be done in the trauma patient to keep urine output > 50 ml/hr.

- For most situations, Ringer's lactate solution or normal saline are adequate fluids to resuscitate the trauma patient.

- These can be given as rapid infusions over 15-20 minute until urine output is within the normal range.

- If urine output remains low even after 4 liters of fluid, blood products should be considered in the resuscitative effort.

Examination of Vital Functions

- Following revival, the trauma patient should be closely examined from head to toe.

- Vital functions and a brief neurological exam should also be performed.

- The **Glasgow coma scale** is useful in determining neurological injury.

THE GLASGOW COMA SCALE

Eyes	Verbal	Motor
1. Do not open	1. Makes no sounds	1. Does not move
2. Open to pain	2. Makes incomprehensible sounds	2. Decerebrate posture (arms in the extended posture)
3. Open to voice	3. Speaks inappropriate words	3. Decorticate posture (arms in the flexed posture)
4. Open spontaneously	4. Confused	4. Withdraws from pain
	5. Alert and oriented	5. Localizes painful stimulus
		6. Obeys commands

Definitive treatment

• The definitive treatment depends on determining a diagnosis. The diagnosis can be established with the following studies:

Radiographic films

• Lateral cervical spine
• AP chest x-ray
• Pelvic film
• Additional films may be required if cervical injury is suspected
  • Lateral spine
  • AP spine
  • Open mouth odontoid

Diagnostic peritoneal lavage (DPL)

• DPL is indicated if abdominal hemorrhage is suspected.
• DPL does not evaluate retroperitoneal organs.

CT-scan

• CT-Scan is a sensitive study in evaluation of the entire abdomen, including retroperitoneal organs; however, it can miss small bowel injuries.
• The surgeon is obligated to rule out intrabdominal injury in the intoxicated or head-injured patient by DPL or CT-scan.

FLUIDS AND ELECTROLYTES

General

- Total body water (**TBW**) is about 60% of body weight.

  - Total body water is higher in adult males and newborns and lower in adult females and obese adults.

- The diagram below indicates the distribution of ions between the intracellular fluid (**ICF**) and extracellular fluid (**ECF**) compartments.

  - The ECF comprises the interstitial fluid and plasma, both of which contain approximately the same ionic composition. However, plasma contains proteins (P)—albumin and globulins—that are not found in the interstitium. The blood (plasma + cells) volume is usually 7% of body weight, i.e., a 70-kg individual has approximately (.07 X 70 = 4.9) 5 liters of blood.

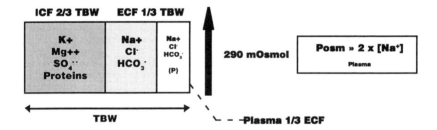

- Na^+ is the principal solute of the extracellular space. It acts to hold water in this compartment.

- Regulation of volume in the intracellular and extracellular compartments occurs via different homeostatic mechanisms:

  - **Plasma osmolality** plays the primary role in the regulation of **intracellular volume**. This is achieved by **homeostasis of water**. This is important for normal cellular functioning.

  - **Plasma Na^+** plays the primary role in the regulation of **plasma volume**. Thus, Na^+ homeostasis is essential for **tissue perfusion**.

- Regulation of plasma osmolality and regulation of Na^+ respond to different signals, are sensed by different receptors, and act on different effectors.

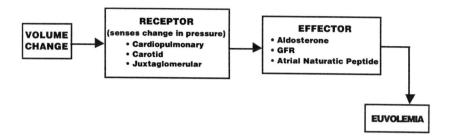

- The primary aim of the effectors is to affect Na^+ reabsorption or secretion by the kidney.

    - ↑ **volume → atrial natriuretic peptide → ↑ Na^+ secretion → EUVOLEMIA**

    - ↓ **volume → aldosterone → ↑ Na^+ reabsorption → EUVOLEMIA**

- The sensors for osmolality are located in the hypothalamus and respond to small changes in plasma osmolality to keep it at a narrow window between 275-290 mOsmol.

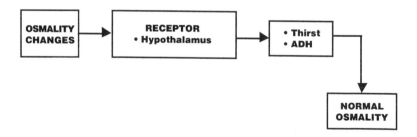

- Persistent hyposmolality and hyponatremia rarely occur due to the ability of the kidney to excrete 10-20 liters of water per day. Hyposmolality may be seen in patients with renal impairment or patients who are comatose.

- Homeostatic regulation of volume and osmolality can occur independently or concurrently to restore volume and osmolality.

    A. A patient who receives an infusion of an isotonic saline responds to volume changes but not to osmolality changes. This patient compensates for volume increase by releasing **atrial natriuretic peptide (ANP)** resulting in increased secretion of Na^+ by the kidney. Because osmolality has not been altered, neither thirst nor ADH secretion is activated.

B. A patient who receives an infusion of hypotonic saline responds both by volume and osmolality changes. The increase in volume results in Na^+ secretion. The hyposmolality induced by hypotonic saline suppresses ADH and thirst resulting in excretion of water into the urine.

Surgical causes of volume depletion

* Volume depletion occurs when output cannot be compensated by input.

* The following are common causes of volume depletion:

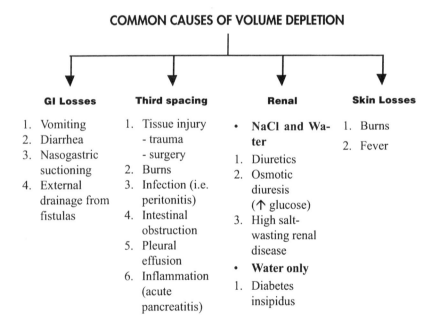

COMMON CAUSES OF VOLUME DEPLETION

GI Losses

1. Vomiting
2. Diarrhea
3. Nasogastric suctioning
4. External drainage from fistulas

Third spacing

1. Tissue injury
   - trauma
   - surgery
2. Burns
3. Infection (i.e. peritonitis)
4. Intestinal obstruction
5. Pleural effusion
6. Inflammation (acute pancreatitis)

Renal

* **NaCl and Water**
1. Diuretics
2. Osmotic diuresis ($\uparrow$ glucose)
3. High salt-wasting renal disease

* **Water only**
1. Diabetes insipidus

Skin Losses

1. Burns
2. Fever

Gastrointestinal losses

- GI losses occur frequently in the surgical patient. These abnormalities are recognized because they are often associated with acid-base disturbances.

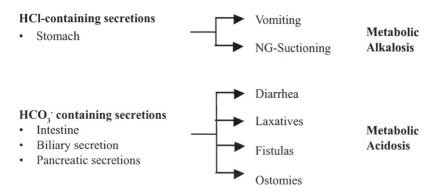

HCl-containing secretions
- Stomach

Vomiting

NG-Suctioning

Metabolic Alkalosis

HCO_3^- containing secretions
- Intestine
- Biliary secretion
- Pancreatic secretions

Diarrhea

Laxatives

Fistulas

Ostomies

Metabolic Acidosis

- GI losses can also occur due to blood loss; however, these do not produce fluid and electrolyte abnormalities.

Third Spacing

- **Third spacing** is the loss of fluid from the intravascular space leading to accumulation in the interstitium or body cavities. After a fractured hip, for example, a patient may accumulate 1.5-2.0 liters of fluid in the interstitium.

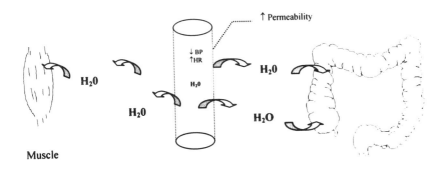

↑ Permeability

↓ BP
↑ HR

H_2O

H_2O

H_2O

H_2O

H_2O

Muscle

- The rate of fluid loss is important. Only those losses for which Na^+ concentration have been unable to compensate for the fluid loss are considered to be third spacing fluid loss.

- A patient with ascites presents with edema instead of volume depletion because the intravascular fluid lost into the peritoneal cavity occurs over a long period of time, resulting in Na^+ compensation. Thus, ascites is not considered to be third spacing.

Renal losses

- Renal losses can occur in the setting of water and salts or water only;
  - Water and salt losses:
    1. Diuretics
    2. Osmotic diuresis (diabetes mellitus)
    3. Adrenal insufficiency
    4. Nephropaty
  - Water losses
    1. Diabetes insipidus
       A. Central
       B. Nephrogenic

Skin losses

- In the surgical patient most significant skin losses are due to burns. The lost fluid has the same ionic composition as plasma.

Clinical manifestations

- The clinical manifestations of volume depletion depend on three parameters:
  1. The manner of fluid loss (i.e., bleeding vs. vomiting)
  2. Electrolyte abnormalities (i.e., hyponatremia ⑧ lethargy, confusion)
  3. Decreased perfusion
- The clinical manifestation of fluid depletion are primarily due to volume depletion in the intravascular space, which results in **hemodynamic manifestations** such as heart rate and blood pressure changes. This is due to the sympathetic compensation that follows volume depletion to maintain appropriate perfusion. There are two main mechanisms of compensation:
  - Vascular:
    - " HR, " vascular resistance to nonvital organs (intestinal), " contractility and cardiac output
  - Endocrine:
    - Angiotesin II
- These mechanisms usually lead to adequate tissue perfusion in the case of mild volume depletion, but cannot completely compensate for moderate or severe cases, which results in the clinical manifestations observed.

- Volume depletion in the interstitial compartments may manifest as changes in **tissue turgor**.

- History and physical examination in a patient with fluid deficits is most useful in trying to determine the magnitude of fluid loss. Patients can be roughly categorized into three groups of dehydration (mild, moderate, and severe) based on history, physical examination and some laboratory data.

- The clinical manifestations related to the magnitude of fluid loss are summarized in the table below:

Magnitude of fluid loss	Signs	Symptoms	Laboratory findings
Mild *10% ECF loss*	Thirst Mildly decreased urine output	Usually none	↑ urine sp. gravity
Moderate *20% ECF loss*	Drowsiness	Decreased skin turgor	↑↑ urine sp. gravity
·	Apathy	Dry mucous membranes	↑ Hct.
·	Decreased urine output	Tachycardia Hypotension	↑ BUN/Cr ratio > 20:1
Severe *30% ECF loss*	Stupor Coma Anuria	Pale, cyanotic, cool skin Sunken eyes Weak pulse Hypotension	↑↑ Hct. ↑↑ BUN/Cr ratio

Management

- The management of a patient with volume depletion begins by ensuring that the patient is hemodynamically stable. Volume assessment is part of the "C" in the "ABC" (airway, breathing, circulation) mnemonic used in resuscitation.

- Following assessment of hemodynamic stability, an adequate history should be taken to try to determine the cause of volume depletion. The common causes outlined above may guide the history taking to try to assess the nature of fluid loss.

- A good physical examination should be conducted to attempt to assess the magnitude of fluid loss.

- Orthostatic blood pressure measurements should be performed on any patient suspected to be volume depleted.
  - Weight change is a valuable parameter if previous values are known.

- Decrease in volume occurs primarily in the venous system. Thus, assessment of JVP is an accurate predictor of volume depletion.

- Determination of urinary Na^+ is also important in establishing the presence of volume depletion.

- The most important parameter to establish volume depletion is urinary $Na^+ < 20$ meq/ L. This is only true in the absence of renal disease.

> **Urinary Na^+ < 20 meq/L = Inadequate tissue perfusion**

- Urine output is also a good predictor of the degree of volume depletion. Normal urine output is > 30 ml/hr and >50 ml/hr in the trauma patient.

- It is important, however, to differentiate between the various causes of decreased urine output (oliguria).

- Oliguric renal failure is defined as urine output < 400 ml/day.

- Oliguria is divided into three categories:

÷ **Postrenal azotemia**: Oliguria caused by obstruction of the urinary system below the kidneys.

- Common causes include:

  - nephroliathisis, benign prostatic hyperplasia causing obstruction, or penile strictures.

This type of azotemia should be excluded first by insertion of a Foley catheter and ultrasound (ultrasound may reveal hydronephrosis = distension of the urinary collecting system by fluid). Once postrenal azotemia has been excluded, an important distinction of azotemia in the surgical patient is the difference between prerenal and postrenal azotemia.

÷ **Prerenal azotemia**: Oliguria caused by decreased renal perfusion. Common causes include: hypotension (e.g., shock), cardiac causes (e.g., severe CHF), severe volume depletion, or bleeding. Drugs that may exacerbate prerenal azotemia include: NSAIDS, ACE inhibitors, or diuretics. BUN/Cr ratio is usually > 20:1, urinary Na^+ excretion is usually less than 10 to 15 meq/liter.

÷ **Renal azotemia**: Oliguria caused by pathology to the functional units of the kidney, which include some glomerulonephropathies and acute tubular necrosis (ATN). Renal azotemia is primarily caused by ATN.

The distinction between prerenal and renal azotemia can also be made on the basis of the fractional excretion of sodium **FeNa**, which can be calculated by the following formula:

$$FeNa = \frac{Serum\ Cr\ X\ Urine\ Na}{Serum\ Na\ X\ Urine\ Cr}\ X\ 100$$

A value of less than 1% is indicative of prerenal azotemia, while a value greater than 1% is indicative of renal azotemia.

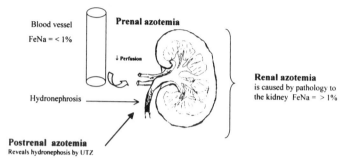

Treatment

- Effective treatment of volume depletion is dependent on correcting the underlying problem leading to the fluid deficit.
- Correction of electrolytes is essential in the management of volume repletion.
- Fluid administration should occur only after the composition of the loss has been established.
- The following table illustrates various fluids used for replenishment:

Fluid	Na+	Cl-	K+	Ca++	Glucose	Lactate
	meq/L	meq/L	meq/L	meq/L	g/l	meq/L
Normal Saline	154	154				
° Normal Saline	77	77				
˜ Normal Saline	39	39				
D₅W						
5% Dextrose/NS					50	
D₅NS						
5% Dextrose/NS	154	154			50	
Ringer's Lactate	130	109	4.0	3.0		28

- Isotonic fluid losses should be corrected by IV administration of Ringer's lactate or normal saline.

- The rate of infusion depends on the severity of the fluid loss. If the patient's orthostatic or oliguric, rapid infusion of 1-2 liters of normal saline or Ringer's lactate over 15-30 minutes is appropriate.

- Complete fluid repletion should be accomplished over a 24-hour period.

- **The appropriateness of the management should be determined by close monitoring of hemodynamic values and urine output.**

- Periodic physical exams should assess:

  - Pulmonary auscultation to listen for crackles
  - Cardiac examination to rule out S_3 sound
  - Neck vein distension
  - Peripheral edema

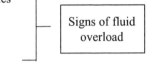
Signs of fluid overload

- Ringer's lactate should be avoided in patients with metabolic alkalosis, as lactate is converted to bicarbonate in the blood stream.

- Fluid replacement should be done carefully on patients with heart disease.

- Volume expander fluids (albumin, hetastarch) are primarily indicated for burns or fluid losses caused by the nephrotic syndrome as well as patients with liver disease.

- **The rate of fluid maintenance can be determined by the general 4/2/1 rule of thumb in which 4 ml/hr are administered for the first 10 Kg, 2 ml/hr for the next 10 and 1 ml/hr for each Kg beyond 20 Kg.**

  i.e. a 70 kg patient:

  4 X 10 kg = 40 ml/hr
  2 X 10 kg = 20 ml/hr
  1 X <u>50 kg = 50 ml/hr</u>
  70 kg   110 ml/hr

Most fluid losses can be corrected by 1/2 NS @ rates 50-100 ml/hr.

Surgical causes of volume excess

- In the surgical patient, a common cause of fluid overload is administration of too much fluid. This is especially worrisome in patients about three days post operatively as fluids return to the intravascular space following **third spacing**.

- Iatrogenic fluid overload also occurs in patients immediately after surgery or trauma as water and sodium excretion is diminished by the kidney. In the absence of intracellular disturbances, this type of fluid overload is isotonic.

- Other forms of fluid overload occur in patients with CHF, oliguric renal failure, and hypoalbuminemia secondary to liver failure. Decreased sodium excretion accounts for the accumulation of excess water.

- Infusion of fluids in the presence of ADH (as occurs in the surgically stressed patient) may lead to isotonic fluid exess.

- Rapid infusion of hyperosmolar substances such as mannitol or contrast materials may lead to hyperosmotic volume execess.

Clinical manifestations/ Signs and symptoms

MILD FLUID OVERLOAD	SEVERE FLUID OVERLOAD
• Weight ↑	• Pulmonary edema
• Hemoglobin/ hematocrit ↓	• Pleural effusions
• ↑ JVP	• Hepatomegaly
• Sacral/ peripheral edema	• Anasarca

Evaluation/management

- History and physical examination (H&P) should be the initial steps in the management to try to assess the nature of the disorder.

- Particular attention should be paid to the heart and lungs to identify evidence of CHF.

- Urinalysis, CBC, and electrolytes with BUN and creatinine should narrow the differential diagnosis.

- Foley catheter insertion is indicated to closely monitor urine output. However, the precise nature of fluid status can be best assessed by central venous pressure (CVP) monitoring. CVP catheter placement is indicated if the fluid status of the patient cannot be assessed by H&P or laboratory analysis.

Treatment

- Mild fluid overload can be successfully treated by fluid and Na^+ restriction.

- More severe cases may require administration of furosemide.

- In case of fluid overload secondary to CHF, cardiotonic drugs and diuretics should help to increase the urine output and correct the disorder.

- It is important to note that intravascular fluid excess is the result of increased total body Na^+.

Surgical causes of hyponatremia

* The most common cause of hyponatremia is excess free water. In the surgical patient this is most often due to elevated levels of ADH.

* Elevated levels of ADH can also be observed in patients with ADH secreting tumors.

* Excess water can also occur secondary to the following underlying diseases:
    - Severe CHF
    - Cirrhosis
    - Neprhotic syndrome

* These conditions are often associated with an edematous state and have decreased effective circulating volume.

* Other forms of excess water occur in the hyperosmolar state. These may be due to:
    - Untreated hyperglycemia.
    - Infusion of active solutes such as mannitol.

* **Pseudohyponatremia** occurs when elevated levels of lipids or protein in the serum result in falsely decreased levels of Na^+ in the plasma. This condition does not produce signs or symptoms of hyponatremia.

Clinical manifestations

The clinical manifestations of hyponatremia are primarily neurological:
* Nausea and Vomiting
* Lethargy
* Confusion
* Seizures
* Coma

Treatment

* The treatment of hyponatremia depends on the severity and the rate of Na^+ loss.
* Patients with hypovolemic hyponatremia are symptomatic primarily due to volume depletion. Re-establishing euvolemia should be the form of treatment for these patients.

- In the hyponatremic patient without symptoms who is either euvolemic or hypervolemic, simple water restriction should be the only form of treatment.

Surgical Causes of Hypernatremia

- In the surgical patient hypernatremia is less common.
- Hypernatremia occurs when water loss is greater than solute loss. This can occur when there are large insensitive losses as may occur in a patient with a tracheostomy breathing humidified air. Vomiting, diarrhea and burns also account for water loss and may result in hyponatremia.

Clinical manifestations

Clinical manifestations of hypernatremia are primarily neurologic:

- Tremors
- Confusion
- Stupor
- Coma
- Peripheral and pulmonary edema may be secondary to hyperosmolarity

Treatment

- Replete water deficit slowly with D_5W or 1/2 NS
- Water deficit in liters = 0.60 X TBW in kg X [(serum Na^+ mmol/L / 140) – 1]
- Only one half of the water deficit should be corrected over the first 24 hours

Surgical causes of hypokalemia

- Inappropriate intake
  - Insufficient supplementation
- Cell shifts
  - Insulin
  - β-agonists
  - Metabolic alkalosis

- K^+ wasting
  - Gastrointestinal
    - Diarrhea
    - Vomiting
    - NG aspiration
    - Intestinal fistula
  - Renal
    - Diuretics
    - Hyperaldosteronism
    - Amphotericin

Clinical manifestations

- Nausea and vomiting
- Weakness
- Tetany
- Ileus
- Paresthesia
- Arrhythmia

EKG Findings

- U waves
- S T segment depression
- Premature ventricular contractions
- Atrial fibrillation

Treatment

- KCl given either IV or PO. The bioavailability of KCl is essentially equivalent by either route: 10 meq of KCl IV or PO should result in 0.1 meq/L in serum.

Surgical causes of hyperkalemia

- $\leq K^+$ intake
  - Iatrogenic
- Cell shifts
  - Insufficient insulin
  - Metabolic acidosis
  - β-blockers
  - Blood transfusion
  - Tissue injury
- Impaired excretion

- Renal failure
- K⁺-sparing diuretics
- Hypoaldosteronism

Clinical manifestations
- Paresthesias
- Weakness
- Decreased reflexes
- Respiratory failure
- Arrhythmias

EKG Findings
- Peaked T waves
- Bradycardia
- Depressed ST segment
- Prolonged PR
- Widened QRS
- Ventricular fibrillation

Treatment
- Treatment is divided into two steps depending on EKG changes.
    - If there are EKG changes, immediate treatment should be cardioprotection with Ca++ followed by reduction of serum K⁺.
    - If there are no EKG changes, treatment should be targeted at reducing the K⁺, which can be accomplished in various ways:

    1. IV Ca⁺⁺ (cardioprotective)
    2. Shift into cells
        - Insulin and glucose
        - Kayexalate
    3. Elimination of K⁺ from the body
        - Sodium polystyrene sulfonate
        - Furosemide
        - Dialysis (in extremely acute cases)

Surgical causes of hypercalcemia
- The various causes of hypercalcemia are easily remembered by the mnemonic:

CHIMPANZEES

- Calcium = ↑ Ca^{++} uptake (milk alkali syndrome)
- Hyperparathyroidism (1° hyperparathyroidism is associated with ↑ Ca^{++})
- Iatrogenic (drug induced as occurs with thiazides, or lithium)
- Metastasis (bone and prostate metastasis can lead to ↑ Ca^{++})
- Paget's disease of bone
- Addison's disease
- Neoplasm as in metastasis
- Zollinger-Ellison syndrome (MEN I - 1° HPT)
- Excessive vitamin D intake
- Excessive vitamin A intake
- Sarcoidosis

Clinical Manifestations

- Mild hypercalcemia is usually asymptomatic.
- Chronic hypercalcemia as it occurs with hyperparathyroidism may present with bone disease and nephrolithiasis.
- The signs and symptoms of acute hypercalcemia include:
  - **General**: weakness, dehydration
  - **Neurologic**: altered mental status
  - **Cardiac**: QT shortening, arrhythmias
  - **Gastrointestinal**: nausea, vomiting, constipation, adynamic ileus

Treatment

- Mild hypercalcemia is treated by ↓ PO intake of Ca++.
- Chronic hypercalcemia mandates a workup to investigate the source of the ↑ Ca^{++}.
- Acute hypercalcemia may be treated as follows:
  - Aggressive diuresis → volume repletion followed by diuresis is the mainstay of treatment.
  - Furosemide
  - Calcitonin
  - Pamidronate disodium

Clinical causes of hypocalcemia

- Vitamin D deficiency
- Hypomagnesemia
- Surgery (Neck surgery)

- Calcium sequestration:
    - acute pancreatitis
    - intestinal bypass surgery
    - short bowel syndrome
    - sepsis
    - rhabdomyolysis

Clinical Manifestations:

- Neurologic
    - confusion
    - parathesias
    - Chvostek's sign = facial muscle spasm with tapping of facial nerve
    - seizures
    - ↑ DTRs
    - tetany
- Psychiatric
    - depression
    - paranoia
- Abdominal cramps
- Cardiac
    - prolonged QT segment
    - arrhythmias

Treatment

- Correct serum Ca^{++} concentration is serum albumin is low.
- Replete with calcium gluconate.

Surgical causes of hypermagnesemia

- Usually iatrogenic as in TPN and IV over-supplementation
- Renal failure

Clinical Manifestations

- Depression of voluntary muscles
    - respiratory depression
- ↓ DTRs
- Cardiac
    - hypotension

Treatment

- Discontinue exogenous Mg^{++} supplementation
- Calcium gluconate
- Hydration
- Furosemide
- Dialysis

Surgical Causes of hypomagnesemia

- Gastrointestinal loss
  - GI suctioning
  - diarrhea
  - vomiting
  - malabsorption
  - biliary fistulas
- Renal losses
  - renal tubular acidosis (RTA)
- Drugs
  - loop diuretics
  - aminoglycosides
  - cisplatin

Clinical Manifestations

- Neuromuscular
  - ↑ DTRs
  - tetany
  - tremor
  - Chvostek's sign
- Cardiac
  - arrhythmias
  - tachycardia
  - ventricular ectopy

Treatment

- PO → Magnesium oxide
- $MgSO_4$ IV

Acid/Base Disturbances

General

- It is important to verify the accuracy of laboratory values whenever an acid base disturbance is encountered. This is accomplished by use of the Henderson Equation:

$$[H+nM] = 24 \times \frac{pCO_2 \text{ (mmHg)}}{[HCO_3^-] \text{ (meq/L)}}$$

- Once the laboratory values have been computed into this equation and they do not validate it, a new set of labs should be obtained.
- Acid-Base disturbances which are seen in the blood are referred to as acidemia/alkalemia. However, the primary disturbance is called acidosis/alkalosis.

Metabolic Acidosis

- Metabolic acidosis is categorized in terms of anion gap:

  Anion Gap $= Na^+ - (Cl^- + HCO_3^-)$
- Normal anion gap varies according to the instruments used by the hospital and is usually referred to as the delta (D) value. The degree of deviation from the standard value is conventionally termed delta-delta (DD value).

Surgical Causes of Metabolic Acidosis

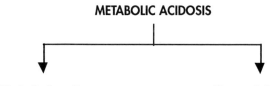

METABOLIC ACIDOSIS

High Anion Gap

MUP PILES

- Methanol
- Uremia
- DKA
- Paraldehyde
- Isopropanol
- Lactic acid
- Ethylene glycol
- Salicylate

Normal Anion Gap

- **Hyperchloremic**

  1. RTA
  2. K^+-Sparing diuretics
  3. Hypoaldosteronism
- **Normal Chloride**

  1. Diarrhea
  2. Carbonic anhydrase inhibitors

Clinical Manifestations:

- Low pH and low HCO_3^-
- Respiratory compensation:
  - The measured pCO_2 should be consistent with the expected compensation.
  - The expected compensation can be calculated by the following relationship:

$pCO_2 =$ $1.5 \times [HCO_3^-] + (8 \pm 2)$	Measured $pCO_2 >$ expected pCO_2	Respiratory alkalosis
	Measured $pCO_2 <$ expected pCO_2	Respiratory acidosis

- Certain causes of anion gap metabolic acidosis are associated with specific clinical manifestations:

Methanol	Retinal changes, ($\uparrow$ osmolar gap)
DKA	Breath, ketones in the urine
Lactic Acid	Malignancy, bowel necrosis
Ethylene glycol	Oxalate crystals in the urine, ($\uparrow$ osmolar gap)
Salicylate	Respiratory alkalosis

- Normal anion gap metabolic acidosis may be caused by renal tubular acidosis (RTA):

Type of RTA	Defect	Clinical Manifestations
Distal RTA **Type I**	Inability of the distal tubule to secrete H^+	• Urine pH > 5.5 even with acid challenge • Associated with: - $\uparrow$ urinary Ca^{++} - Urolithiasis - Osteomalacia • $\downarrow K^+$
Proximal RTA **Type II**	Inability of the proximal tubule to reabsorb HCO_3^-	• Urine pH < 5.5 • $\downarrow K^+$ • Sometimes Fanconi's syndrome
Type IV RTA	$\downarrow$aldosterone $\downarrow$renin	• $\uparrow K^+$ • history of diabetes

Treatment

- The goal of treatment should be directed toward treatment of the underlying disease causing the acidosis. In most cases this simply involves removal of an offending agent (e.g., methanol, acetazolamide).
- HCO_3^- can be administered in severe cases of metabolic acidosis. A small amount of HCO_3^- can correct RTA I, but not RTA II.

Metabolic Alkalosis

Surgical Causes of Metabolic Alkalosis

- The etiology of metabolic alkalosis can be divided based on chloride responsiveness.

Chloride Resistant	Chloride Responsive
1. Primary aldosteronism	1. Diuretic use
2. High renin state	2. Post hypercapnic alkalosis
3. Cushing's disease	3. Vomiting and gastric suctioning
4. Bartter's syndrome	

Clinical Manifestations

- high HCO_3^-, high pH
- respiratory response:
  - $\rightarrow pCO_2 = 0.9 \times [HCO_3^-] + 9 \pm 2$
  - $\rightarrow$ for each meq - HCO_3^-, pCO_2 - 0.5 mmHg
- weakness
- tetany
- cardiovascular instability
- " lactate production

Treatment

Chloride Resistant	Chloride Responsive
1. Treat the source of aldosterone	1. Treat underlying disorder
2. Treat renal artery stenosis	2. Hydration (NS)
3. May use Ca^{++} channel blockers	3. KCl replacement

Respiratory Alkalosis

General

- Respiratory disorders are classified as acute or chronic.
- The hallmark of chronic respiratory processes is the HCO_3^- compensation. The kidney takes up to two days to compensate for respiratory disturbances. If the HCO_3^- is normal, the respiratory process is most likely acute.

Surgical Causes of Respiratory Acidosis

- Respiratory depression
    - drugs
    - organic disease
- Neuromuscular disorders
- Cardiopulmonary arrest

Clinical Manifestations

- High pCO_2, low pH
- Metabolic compensation
    Acute: HCO_3^- - 0.1 meq/L for each 1 mmHg - in pCO_2
    Chronic: HCO_3^- - 0.3 meq/L for each 1 mmHg - in pCO_2

Treatment

- Diagnose and treat underlying problems.

Respiratory Acidosis

Surgical Causes of Respiratory Acidosis

- Acute of Chronic hyperventilation
    - Acute hypoxia
        - pneumonia
        - bronchospasm
        - pulmonary edema
    - Chronic hypoxia
        - heart disease
        - anemia
    - Respiratory center stimulation
        - aspirin intoxication
        - anxiety
        - fever

Clinical Manifestations

- Low pCO_2, high pH
- Metabolic compensation
    Acute: HCO_3^- ↓0.1 meq/L for each 1 mmHg ↓in pCO_2
    Chronic: HCO_3^- ↓0.3 meq/L for each 1 mmHg ↓in pCO_2

Treatment

- Diagnose and treat underlying disease.

Mixed Acid-Base Disturbances

- More than two acid base disturbances (and sometimes three) can often be encountered in the surgical patient.
- It is important to delineate the degree of compensation expected, keeping in mind that compensatory mechanisms never bring the system completely back to normal.
- In mixed metabolic acidosis/alkalosis the Delta-delta value can delineate the presence of a combined disturbance (see chart below).

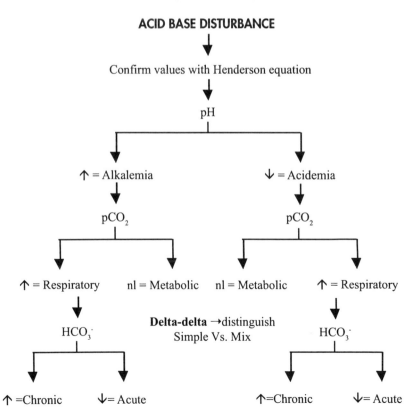

2 | PEDIATRIC SURGERY

Congenital Pediatric Conditions

- The majority of general pediatric disorders requiring surgery fall into the congenital category.
- The following are the common congenital disorders affecting newborns and children.

Neck	Thorax	Abdomen
1. Dermoid cyst	1. Esophageal atresia/ Tracheoesophageal fistula	1. Congenital pyloric stenosis
2. Thyroglossal duct cyst		2. Intestinal atresia
3. Pharyngeal cleft cyst	2. Congenital diaphragmatic hernia (CDH)	3. Hirschprung's disease
4. Cystic hygroma		4. Omphalocele
		5. Gastrochisis
		6. Biliary atresia
		7. Choledochal cysts
		8. Anorectal malformations
		9. Necrotizing enterocolititis (NEC)
		10. Hernias
		11. Undescended testis
		12. Malrotation of intestine
		13. Meckcl's diverticulum

Congenital Masses of the Neck

General

- These masses are characteristically soft, painless and persistent and occur early in life.
  - Location and characteristics can distinguish the various types of congenital masses commonly encountered.
  - The following are common congenital masses:

  1. Dermoid cyst (DC)
     - Dermoid cysts occur due to a defect in the fusion of somatic segments.
     - Accumulation of sebaceous secretions lead to swelling.
     - **These masses usually occur in the midline of the neck.**
  2. Thyroglossal duct cyst (TDC)
     - These occur due to remnants of the thyroid diverticulum during its migration from the base of the tongue (foramen cecum) to the normal position of the thyroid gland.
     - Accumulation of mucus may lead and swelling and infection.
     - Move up and down with swallowing
     - **These masses also occur in the midline of the neck.**
  3. Pharyngeal cleft sinus (PCS)
     - These are remnants of pharyngeal clefts.
     - **These masses usually occur in the anterolateral aspect of the neck.**
  4. Cystic hygroma (CH)
     - Cystic Hygromas occur when there is obliteration of lymphatic drainage.
     - These masses are present at the time of birth.
     - **These masses are commonly located in the posterior aspect of the sternocleidomastoid muscle.**

Clinical Manifestations

- These masses are present at birth
- Soft, and painless
- These masses may obstruct the trachea and/or esophagus and present with:
  - stridor
  - dyspnea
  - dysphagia

Treatment

- Surgical removal is indicated for the management of these neck masses.
- TDC should be treated by removal of the cyst trunk and hyoid bone at the mid-point to avoid recurrence (Sistrunk procedure).

Congenital Conditions of the Thorax

Esophageal Atresia/ Tracheoesophageal Fistula

General

- Esophageal atresia occurs when there is incomplete development of the esophagus, which results in the formation of a blind-ending esophagus.

- Formation of fistulas with the trachea are common and may occur with the distal and/or the proximal segment of the incomplete esophagus.

- In about 10% of the cases, esophageal atresia and TE fistula may be associated with other congenital abnormalities. These abnormalities called the VACTER cluster (Vertebral, Anal, Cardiac, Tracheal, Esophageal, Radial and Renal). Finding of one abnormality mandates investigation for other abnormalities in this cluster.

- There are five possible combinations which occur with different degrees of frequency.

1%

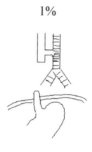

Esophageal atresia with proximal tracheoesophageal fistula

2%

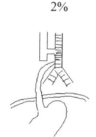

Esophageal atresia with proximal and distal tracheoesophageal fistula

4%

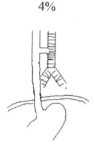

Tracheoesophageal fistula without atresia

8%

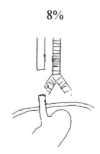

Esophageal atresia without tracheoesophageal fistula

85%

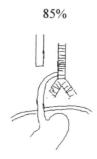

Esophageal atresia with distal tracheoesophagcal fistula

Diagnosis

- The diagnosis is made based on H&P, NG-tube, abdominal and chest x-rays.

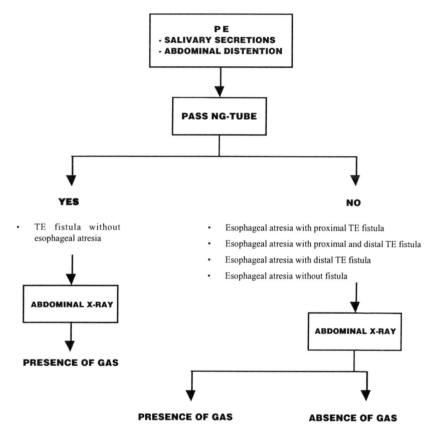

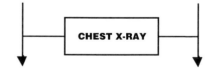

Treatment
- Aspiration prevention
    - Place child in the upright position
    - NG suctioning
    - Aspiration antibiotics
- Surgical repair is the definitive treatment

Congenital Diaphragmatic Hernia (CDH)

General
- CDH is an urgent pediatric condition that occurs due to inappropriate development of the diaphragm resulting in herniation of abdominal organs into the thoracic cavity.
- Two sites of the diaphragm are commonly affected:

---

1. BOCHDALEK
- Occurs in the posterolateral aspect of the diaphragm.
- This is the most common type of hernia occurring in 85% of all CDH.
- Occurs more often on the left

2. MORGAGNI
- Occurs in the retrosternal portion of the diaphragm.

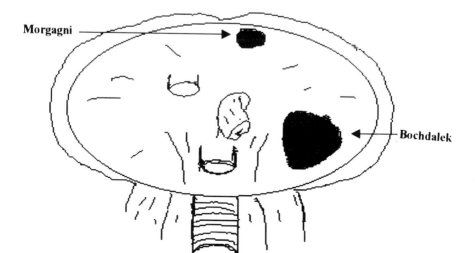

Complications
- Mechanical obstruction of the lungs by herniated viscera.
- Pulmonary hypoplasia
- Persistent pulmonary hypertension

Clinical Manifestations
- Dyspnea
- Cyanosis
- ↓ breath sounds
- Mediastinal deviation
- Heart shift to the right
- Scaphoid abdomen

Diagnosis
- Severe respiratory distress at term birth suggests CDH.
- ↓ Breath sounds and bowel sounds in the chest are highly indicative of CDH.
- Chest x-ray may reveal the presence of air filled loops of bowel in the chest.

Treatment
- Resuscitation
- Endotracheal intubation
- Surgical repair should be done as soon as the newborn is properly resuscitated
- If respiratory distress persists extracorporeal membrane oxygenation (ECMO) is indicated.

ECMO

- Complete respiratory support by cardiopulmonary bypass.

Congenital Conditions of the Abdomen

Congenital Pyloric Stenosis

General
- Pyloric stenosis occurs due to abnormal hypertrophy of the smooth muscle of the pylorus leading to gastric outlet obstruction.
- Risk factors:
    - Male (4:1 Male/Female)
    - Firstborn
    - Family history
    - 2 weeks – 2 months of age

Clinical Manifestations
- A 2 week to 2 month male who presents with **nonbilious projectile vomiting**.
- Vomiting leads to electrolyte abnormalitites: hypokalemia, hypochloremic metabolic alkalosis.
- Urinalysis may reveal paradoxical aciduria as H^+ is secreted in the urine in exchange of K^+.
- If the diagnosis is delayed, weight loss or lack of weight gain may be observed.

Diagnosis
- History and physical examination
    - Physical examination demonstrates an abdominal mass called an **"olive."**
- Electrolyte abnormalities
- Ultrasonography may reveal an elongated pylorus with thickened wall.
- Barium swallow is recommended if the above do not provide a definitive diagnosis.
    - Barium swallow reveals:
        - String sign
        - Double railroad track sign

Treatment
- Prompt correction of fluid and electrolyte abnormalities.
    - Hydration corrects the alkalemia
    - Hypokalemia should be corrected with KCl

- Surgical repair
    - **Pyloromyotomy**
    - Fredet-Ramstedt operation → surgical division of the circular fibers of the smooth muscle without entering the pyloric mucosa.

Duodenal Atresia

General

- Ischemia during development leads to duodenal malformation resulting in stenosis or complete obstruction.
- Other causes of duodenal obstruction include:
    - Annular pancreas
    - Malrotations
- Duodenal atresia is common in newborns with trisomy 21.
- Most newborns with duodenal atresia have associated abnormalities:
    - Other gastrointestinal defects
    - Renal defects
    - Cardiac defects
- Atresia may occur distal (85%) or proximal (15%) to the hepatopancreatic ampulla (of Vater).

Clinical Manifestations

- Distal atresia presents with bilious vomiting and epigastric distension.
- Proximal atresia presents with nonbilious vomiting and epigastric distension.
- Vomiting may lead to fluid and electrolyte abnormalities.

Diagnosis

- History and physical examination
- Abdominal x-ray reveals a **"double-bubble"** sign, one caused by the distended stomach and the other caused by the remaining duodenal segment.

Treatment

- Correction of fluid and electrolyte abnormalities
- Surgical Repair
    - Duodenoduodenostomy
    - Duodenojujenostomy

Jejunal/Ileal Atresia

General

- Jejunal/Ileal atresia or stenosis results in obstruction.
- Other forms of obstruction at the level of the jejunum include:
  - Meconium ileus
  - Intestinal duplication
- Uterovascular accidents are the cause of this congenital defect:
  - Intrauterine volvulus
  - Malrotations
  - Internal hernias
  - Intussusception
- Jujunal or ileal atresias range from simple webs across the lumen of the intestine to multiple atresias.

Clinical Manifestations

- Bilious vomiting
- Abdominal distention
- Failure to pass meconium

Diagnosis

- History and physical examination
- Abdominal x-ray shows multiple air-filled fluid bubbles

Treatment

- Fluid resuscitation
- Surgical resection of the affected area and anastomosis of the bowel.

Hirschprung's Disease

General

- Absence of ganglionic cells in the colonic myenteric (Auerbach's) and submucosal (Meissner's) plexuses results in the lack of peristaltic movements in the affected area, which leads to colonic dilation and functional obstruction.
- This condition is also known as aganglionic (congenital) megacolon.
- Risk Factors:
  - Family history
  - Male gender (4:1 male/female)

- The entire colon is seldom involved. In 80% of cases, the rectum or sigmoid colon is affected.

Clinical Manifestations
- Bilious vomiting
- Abdominal distension
- Weight loss
- Diarrhea
- Constipation
- Failure to pass meconium

Diagnosis
- History and physical examination
    - History of constipation
    - Distended abdomen
- Abdominal x-ray
    - Shows a dilated colon
- Barium enema
    - Reveals a dilated proximal colonic end and a constricted distal end
    - Barium takes much longer to be evacuated
- Biopsy
    - Biopsy is usually performed transanally.
    - Submucosal biopsy is usually sufficient to provide the diagnosis.
    - If the diagnosis is still uncertain, full thickness biopsy should be performed.

Treatment

Surgical correction
- Surgical correction begins with a diverting colostomy in which the distal end of the colon is diverted to the abdominal wall where a surgical defect is created to allow the passage of stool at the affected colonic level (colostomy).
- Several months later, definitive surgery is performed:
- The following surgical procedures are recommended for definitive correction of this defect. They are performed between 6 months and 1 year of life.
    - **Swenson operation**
        - Resection of affected segment and anastomosis to the anus.
    - **Soave operation**
        - This is a "pull through" procedure in which normal colon is brought through the aganglionic rectum which has had its mucosa removed.

- **Duhamel operation**
  - Anastamosis of the anterior affected colon to a posterior portion of unaffected bowel and creation of a functional rectal pouch.

Omphalocele

General

- Omphalocele is a congenital abdominal wall defect that results from failure of closure of abdominal folds during development. The abdominal defect occurs at the umbilical ring and causes abdominal contents (including the liver in many cases) to protrude externally.
- A sac covers the extruded viscera.
- Omphalocele is associated with a high incidence of many other abnormalities including chromosomal abnormalities.
- Omphalocele is part of the Cantred pentand of abnormalities which include:
  - Cardiac defects
  - Diaphragmatic hernia
  - Omphalocele
  - Pericardial abnormalities
  - Sternal cleft

Diagnosis
- The diagnosis is made by prenatal ultrasonography.

Complications
- Malrotation of the gut
- Fluid and heat loss
- Infection

Management
- Prevent heat and fluid losses by covering the extruded intestines with a wet sterile gauze
- NG-tube suctioning
- IV fluid resuscitation
- Broad spectrum antibiotics
- Surgical repair

Gastroschisis

General
- Gastroschisis is a congenital abdominal wall defect that results due to failure of abdominal folds to close during development. This abdominal defect occurs lateral to umbilical ring with higher frequency on the left side. This defect also causes abdominal contents to protrude externally. The liver is not usually involved in this abnormality.
- The extruded viscera are not contained in a sac.
- Unlike omphalocele, the only associated defect is intestinal atresia.

Complications
- Inflamed peritoneum
- Malrotation
- Loss of fluids and heat
- Infection
- Ileus

Management
- Fluid resuscitation
- NG-tube suctioning
- Covering of the extruded bowel with soaked gauze
- Surgical repair

Biliary atresia

General
- Biliary atresia is the obliteration of the biliary hepatic ducts.
- The entire bilary tree is most commonly affected by this condition, but occasionally only a portion is affected.

Clinical Manifestations
- Persistent **jaundice > 2** weeks caused by direct > indirect bilirubin.
- Self-limiting jaundice that resolves within the first two weeks of life is called physiologic jaundice and is caused by inappropriate conjugation of bilirubin by glucuronyl transferase.
- Hepatosplenomegaly
- Portal hypertension → ascites
- Biluria
- Light-colored stools

Differential Diagnosis

- Neonatal infections
    - TORCH (**To**xoplasma, **R**ubella, **C**ytomegalovirus, **H**erpex simplex)
- Neonatal hepatitis
- $\alpha\text{-}_1$-antitrypsin deficiency
- Galactosemia
- Crigler-Najjar syndrome
- Gilbert's syndrome
- Hemolysis

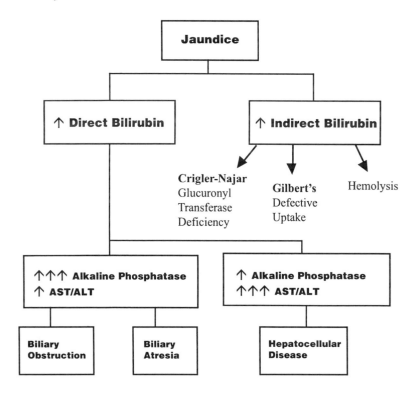

Diagnosis

- The diagnosis of biliary atresia must be made early as the complications with surgical intervention increase with age.
- History and physical examination
    - Persistent jaundice suggests biliary atresia
- Ultrasonography

- HIDA scan
- Intraoperative cholangiogram
- Liver biopsy

Treatment
- Early surgical intervention by the **Kasai procedure**
- The Kasai procedure is the anastamosis of the micoscropic porta hepatis bile ducts to the small bowel.

Choledochal Cyst

General
- Choledochal cyst is the dilatation of the bile ducts with distal obstruction.
- Infants with this condition have an increased risk for the development of choloangiocarcinoma.
- Several types of choledochal cyst are differentiated by the anatomic variant present.

Clinical Manifestations
- Intermittent jaundice
- RUQ mass
- Abdominal pain
- Pancreatitis

Diagnosis
- History and physical examination
- Ultrasonography

Treatment
- Surgical repair with resection of the cyst and a Roux-en-Y hepatojejunostomy.

Anorectal Malformations

General
- Anorectal malformations include the following disorders:
    - Anal atresia
    - Imperforate anus
    - Rectal atresia
- Imperforate anus is the absence of a normal anus.
- The anus may occur at a different location and may form fistulas
- Imperforate anus is subdivided into high and low variants:

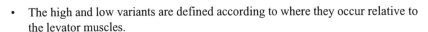
- The high and low variants are defined according to where they occur relative to the levator muscles.
- High abnormalities are more common in males and low malformations are more common in females.
- Imperforate anus is associated with the group of disorders known as the **VACTER** cluster (vertebral, anal, cardiac, tracheal, esophageal, radial and renal).

Clinical Manifestations
- Inspection during physical exam reveals the absence of a normal anus and/or fistulas to the skin.
- Fistulas to the bladder or urethra present with fecaluria and UTIs.
- Fistulas to the vagina.
- Bladder or urethral fistulas may lead to electrolyte abnormalities (hyperchloremic acidosis) as the colon absorbs Cl⁻ from the bladder.

Diagnosis
- Physical examination
- Abdominal x-ray
- Perineal ultrasound

Treatment
- Treatment of high anomalies consists of dilation of the anal fistula and anoplasty.
- Low anomalies are treated with a diverting colostomy. A neoanus is then created about the age of one year.

Necrotizing Enterocolitis (NEC)

General
- NEC is intestinal hemorrhagic mucosal necrosis that may progress to become transmural and involve the entire bowel.
- Transmural involvement may progress to cause shock sepsis and death.
- This is the most common indication for laparotomy in the neonate.
- Risk factors include:
- Prematurity
    - Other debilitating illness (cyanotic heart disease, PDA etc.)
    - Shock
    - Hypoxia
    - Respiratory distress syndrome
- The etiology of NEC is multifactorial and may include:
    - Mucosal ischemia

- Bacterial infection
- Food source for bacterial infection

Clinical Manifestations
- Bloody diarrhea
- Abdominal distension
- Lethargy
- Fever
- Vomiting
- Sepsis
- Jundice
- Abdominal wall erythema

Diagnosis
- Physical examination
- Abdominal x-ray may reveal:
    - Dilated intestinal loops (ileus)
    - Pneumatosis intestinalis (gas within the bowel wall)
    - Free air in the abdomen
    - Portal vein air
- Peritoneal tap
    - Indications for peritoneal tap include:
        - abdominal erythema
        - firm and distended abdomen
        - thrombocytopenia

Treatment
- Most cases of NEC are treated medically:
    - Fluid resuscitation
    - Feeding cessation
    - NG-tube decompression
- Indications for laparotomy include:
    - Transmural perforation or transmural bowel necrosis
    - Distended rigid abdomen
    - Severe thrombocytopenia
    - Abdominal wall erythema
    - Peritoneal tap indicating the presence of bacteria
    - Failure to improve with medical treatment

Acquired Pediatric Conditions

Hernias

General

- An abdominal hernia is the protrusion of any organ (or portion of it) or a structure through an abdominal wall defect, which may be congenital, acquired or iatrogenic.
- The most common type of pediatric hernias is an indirect inguinal hernia.

Hernia type	Male	Female	Children
Direct	40%	Rare	Rare
Indirect	50%	70%	**100%**
Femoral	10%	30%	Rare

- **Indirect Inguinal Hernia**
  - It is a hernia that protrudes through the internal inguinal ring.
  - It contains a sac (processus vaginalis and peritoneum).
  - It is a congenital hernia in that patency of the processus vaginalis is required but not sufficient for its formation.
  - During development there is complete obliteration of the processus vaginalis, which provides direct communication between the scrotum and the peritoneal cavity.
  - Indirect inguinal hernias occur most commonly on the right

- **Direct Inguinal Hernia**
  - It is a hernia that protrudes through the Hasselbach's triangle
  - It occurs lateral to the inferior epigastric vessels.
  - It contains no sac.
  - This type of hernia occurs due to weakening of the abdominal wall.
  - This type of hernia is most common in older adults.

Clinical Manifestations

- Most hernias present as an intermittent mass that appears in the groin.
- There is occasional discomfort and pain with the mass.
- It is often possible to reproduce the symptoms of a hernia by voluntarily increasing abdominal pressure as in the Valsalva maneuver or coughing.

Diagnosis

- The diagnosis of a hernia is primarily made by physical examination.

Treatment

- Any hernia has the potential of incarceration or strangulation. Therefore, surgical repair is recommended at the time of the diagnosis.

Hydrocele

- Failure of obliteration of the processus vaginalis may result in the formation of hydroceles.
- A hydrocele is a sac filled with fluid around the testicle.
- There are two types of hydroceles that can occur:
  - Communicating hydrocele
    - It is a hydeocele that communicates with the peritoneal cavity.
    - Thus, the size of this hydrocele can vary.
  - Noncommunicating hydrocele.
    - Has no communication with the peritoneal cavity
    - The size of this hydrocele remains constant
- A guide test to differentiate between hydrocele and inguinal hernia is to use a flashlight. A hydrocele is more translucent than a hernia.

Acute Appendicitis

General

- Appendicitis occurs due to inflammation of the vermiform appendix caused by narrowing of its lumen.
- Narrowing may be caused by hyperplasia of the appendix (commonly seen in children) or by accumulation of inspissated fecal material (fecalith, commonly seen in young adults).
- Acute appendicitis is the most common cause of acute abdomen.
- The age of onset is classically between 5-35 years old.
- In younger and older patients, the signs and symptoms of appendicitis are more insidious, which results in a higher rate of perforation in these groups.

Clinical Manifestations

- History
  - Pain beginning in the periumbilical region and subsequently localizing to the right lower quadrant of the abdomen.

- Anorexia (reliable symptom of acute appendicitis).
- Nausea and vomiting following the onset of pain.

• Physical Examination
   - Right lower quadrant tenderness (classically the maximal point of tenderness occurs at McBurney's point, one third of the distance from the anterior iliac spine to the umbilicus).
   - Low grade fever
   - Psoas sign (pain on extension of the right hip)
   - Obturator sign (pain on internal or external rotation of the hip)
   - Rovsing's sign (rebound palpation of the left lower quadrant produces pain in the right lower quadrant)
• The clinical findings of acute appendicitis may be different in patients with a retrocecal appendix, which occurs in 15% of cases.
• Laboratory tests
   - Leukocytosis (12,000-14,000 cells/µL)

Diagnosis

• History and physical examination. The diagnosis of acute appendicitis is a clinical one based on signs and symptoms.
• Leukocytosis is often used in the diagnosis of acute appendicitis. A general rule of thumb consists of making the diagnosis of acute appendicitis if two of the following three elements are present:

---

1. Right lower quadrant abdominal pain (must be present)

2. Good history (including anorexia)

3. Leukocytosis (12,000-14,000 cells/µL)

• Acute Abdominal Series (AAS). If the diagnosis is still uncertain based on history and physical examination, an AAS may rule out a number of causes of abdominal pain present in the differential diagnosis. In 5% of the cases, a fecalith can be observed in plain films. Plain films are also useful in assessing perforation by the presence/absence of free air.
• Urinalysis is helpful in ruling out pyelonephritis.
• Ultrasonography/CT studies are helpful in determining the degree of inflammation beyond the appendix and may assess the presence of other pathology when the diagnosis of appendicitis is still not clear.
• Barium enema is useful in children as it shows no filling of the appendix in acute appendicitis.

Treatment

- ABCs and appropriate resuscitation
- Untreated appendicitis may lead to perforation in less than 24 hours. Therefore, a clinical suspicion of acute appendicitis requires prompt surgical intervention.
- Preoperative antibiotics to cover aerobic (and anaerobic if perforation is suspected) bacteria may be administered.
- Postoperative antibiotics for the first 24h without perforation and for seven days with perforation.
- If perforation is found intraoperatively, the incision should be allowed to close by secondary intention.
- An appendectomy should be performed even in the absence of an inflamed appendix. A 20% negative appendicitis rate is acceptable to prevent the risk of complication if appendicitis is missed.
- An appendectomy can also be performed laparoscopically. This procedure is even more desirable in the female patient when the diagnosis of appendicitis is not clear as gynecologic pathology can be explored.

Meckel's Diverticulum

General
- Meckel's diverticulum is a remnant of the embryonic vitelline duct, which connects the yolk sac to the primitive midgut in the embryo.
- It is the most common congenital anomaly of the small bowel.
- A number of characteristics can be remembered by the rule of 2's.

---

1. It is usually located 2 feet from the ileocecal valve
2. Symptoms develop in 2% of the patients
3. Incidence is 2% of the general population
4. There is a 2:1 male/female ratio
5. Symptoms usually occur before the age of 2

Clinical Manifestations
The clinical presentation is dependent on the number of complications that may occur secondary to a symptomatic Meckel's diverticulum.

- Intestinal hemorrhage, especially in children
- Intestinal obstruction, which may present with abdominal pain, nausea, vomiting
- Inflammation, which presents with abdominal pain similar to acute appendicitis
- Incarcerated/strangulated hernias (Littré's hernia)

Diagnosis

- The diagnosis is made primarily by history and physical examination.
- AAS may rule out other conditions of abdominal pain.
- Barium and radionuclide studies may be required if there is suspicion of bleeding.

Treatment

- Symptomatic Meckel's diverticulum should be resected.
- Indications for resection of an asymptomatic diverticulum found incidentally include:
    - Age of the patient < 40 years-old
    - Presence of inflammation
    - Size > 2 inches long
    - Detection of heterotopic tissue
    - Attached mesodiverticular bands

Intussusception

General

- Intussusception is intestinal obstruction that is caused by insertion of a segment of the intestine into an adjacent segment.
- The most common age of onset is between 4 months to 2 years.

Clinical Presentation

- Intussusception clinically presents with signs and symptoms of obstruction.

Diagnosis

- History and physical examination
- Abdominal x-ray
- Ultrasonography

Treatment

- Air enema
- Barium enema
- If enemas are unsuccessful, laparotomy should be performed.

3 | ABDOMINAL SURGERY

Acute Abdomen

General
- Acute abdomen refers to the severe abdominal pain that brings a patient to the hospital.
- Abdominal pain can be divided into different general categories:

> 1. *Visceral Pain* describes poorly localized, dull, diffuse, deep pain that is usually the result of an insult to an organ.
> 2. *Colicky pain* is characteristically intermittent and it is usually caused by obstruction of hollow viscera.
> 3. *Somatic Abdominal Pain* is usually well localized, sharp, superficial pain caused by irritation of the parietal peritoneum.
> 4. *Referred Pain* occurs as a result of commonly innervated pathways (e.g., biliary colic causes right scapular pain)

- Visceral pain should alert the surgeon to an abdominal problem.

Evaluation of acute abdominal pain
- Evaluation of an acute abdomen begins with a good history and physical examination.
- A through history should elicit the following information about the abdominal pain:
  - **Mode of onset: acute pain may be suggestive of a surgical abdomen, ruptured AAA, or perforated viscus.**
  - **Character: sharp vs. dull (see above).**
  - **Duration: first onset vs. previous episodes - cholelithiasis.**
  - **Frequency**
  - **Location**
  - **Aggravating/ alleviating factors**
- Associated symptoms are also an important element of the history.
- **Anorexia, nausea** and **vomiting** may indicate more serious disease.

Right Upper Quadrant

1. Stomach
   - PUD
   - Perforated ulcer
   - Gastritis
2. Gallbladder
   - **Cholelithiasis**
   - **Choledocholithiasis**
   - **Cholecystitis**
   - **Cholangitis**
3. Pancreas
   - Pancreatitis
4. Liver
   - Hepatic abscess
   - Liver tumors
   - Hepatitis
5. Lungs
   - Pneumonia
   - PE
6. Kidney
   - Pyelonephritis
   - Nephrolithiasis

Left Upper Quadrant

1. Stomach
   - PUD
   - Perforated ulcer
   - Gastritis
   - Reflux
2. Spleen
   - **Rupture**
   - **Abscess**
3. Thoracic
   - Pneumonia
   - PE
   - Dissecting aortic aneurysm
4. Kidney
   - Pyelonephritis
   - Nephrolithiasis
5. Hiatal hernia
6. Trauma
   - Boerhaave's syndrome
   - Mallory-Weiss tear

Right Lower Quadrant

1. Small bowel and appendix
   - SBO
   - Meckel's diverticulum
   - **Appendicitis**
   - Intussusception
2. Pancreatitis
3. Colon
   - Diverticulitis
   - Volvulus
   - Perforated viscus
   - Colon CA
   - IBD
4. Renal
   - UTI
   - Nephrolithiasis
5. Ruptured AAA
6. Gynecologic
   - Ectopic pregnancy
   - PID
   - Mittelschmerz
   - Ovarian torsion/cyst/tumor

Left Lower Quadrant

1. Small bowel and appendix
   - SBO
   - Appendicitis
   - Intussusception
2. Colon
   - **Diverticulitis**
   - **Volvulus**
   - **Perforated viscus**
   - **Colon CA**
   - **IBD**
3. Renal
   - UTI
   - Nephrolithiasis
4. Ruptured AAA
5. Gynecologic
   - Ectopic pregnancy
   - PID
   - Mittelschmerz
   - Ovarian torsion/tumor

Differential Diagnosis

• The differential diagnosis of abdominal pain by quadrant is shown above on page 52:

Physical Examination

This should assess the severity of the disease (i.e. is the patient sick?), estimate the degree of pain, identify areas of maximal pain, and identify non-abdominal causes of pain. The physical examination of the abdomen should include:

• **Inspection**
  - Previous surgical scars - think adhesion - SBO
  - Abdominal distention
• **Auscultation**
  - Bowel sounds - ileus vs. SBO
  - Bruits - AAA
• **Palpation**
  - Voluntary guarding (abdominal muscle contraction with palpation of the abdomen)
  - Involuntary guarding (rigid abdominal muscles even without palpation)
  - Rebound tenderness (pain caused by stretch and release of the inflamed peritoneum)

COMMON SIGNS

• **Murphy's sign** suggests an inflamed gallbladder. Occurs when there is arrest of inspiration with palpation of the right upper quadrant

• **Obturator sign** suggests appendicitis. Occurs when there is suprapubic pain with internal rotation of the hip

• **Psoas sign** suggests appendicitis. Occurs when there is suprapubic pain with extension of the hip

• **Rovsing's sign** suggests appendicitis. Occurs when rebound palpation of the left lower quadrant produces pain in the right lower quadrant

---

  - Costovertebral angle tenderness (CVA-T) is suggestive of pyelonephritis and possibly stone disease.
  - Abdominal pain mandates careful rectal and pelvic examination
  - Exclude hernia
• **Percussion**
  - Assess liver and spleen size

Investigative studies
- CBC with differential
- Electrolytes, BUN, Creatinine
- Amylase
- Urinalysis
- Pregnancy test
- Liver function tests
- X-ray, acute abdominal series, ultrasound, CT-scan, ECG

Working Diagnosis requiring immediate laparotomy
- Ruptured aneurysm
- Ruptured ectopic pregnancy
- Spontaneous splenic or hepatic rupture
- Hemodynamic instability

Working Diagnosis requiring urgent laparotomy
- Perforated viscus
- Appendicitis
- Strangulated hernia
- Mesenteric ischemia
- Bowel obstruction
- Peritoneal signs, sepsis

Treatment
- Treatment of causes of an acute abdomen with an uncertain diagnosis should be targeted at ameliorating the symptoms with pain medication and close observation in the hospital.
- Surgery is indicated when one of the above diagnoses is suspected or when a patient with abdominal trauma deteriorates in spite of aggressive medical management.

- **Pain along with tenderness is almost always suggestive of abdominal pathology requiring surgery.**
- **If these two clinical manifestations are present the surgeon needs a good reason not to operate immediately.**

Gastrointestinal Bleeding

General

• Gastrointestinal bleeding (GI-bleed) is usually classified into upper GI-bleed if it occurs proximal to the ligament of Trietz (located at the junction of duodenum and jejunum) and lower GI-bleed for bleeding distal to the ligament of Trietz.

• Massive GI-bleed is defined as > 8 L/blood loss in 24 hours and this may be an indication for laparotomy.

• After ensuring hemodynamic and patient stability, it is important to establish if the source of bleeding is from the upper or lower GI tract.

• The initial step in identifying the source of bleeding consists of a good history followed by nasogastric (NG)-tube suction, which can usually differentiate between upper or lower GI-bleeding.

  - If NG-tube aspiration is negative, anoscopy/ proctoscopy should be performed.

  - If NG-tube aspiration is positive for blood, upper GI endoscopy should be the next step in identifying the source of bleeding.

Upper GI-Bleeding

Common Causes of Upper GI-bleeding include:

Duodenal ulcer	25%
Gastric ulcer	20%
Acute Gastritis	15%
Mallory-Weiss Tear	10%
Esophageal/Gastric varices	8%

Clinical Manifestations

• Hematemesis (bloody vomit)

• Melena (black, tarry stool)

• Hematochezia (bloody stools) in massive upper GI-bleeding

• Epigastric discomfort

• Weakness

• Syncope, shock

• Guaiac (+) stool

Diagnosis

• Evaluation of GI-bleeding begins with a good history and physical examination.

- CBC with platelets
- PT/PTT
- Type and cross match
- Serum electrolyte values are useful to determine the amount of fluid loss.
- Liver function tests (LFTs)
- Upper GI endoscopy is the test of choice and is especially useful in identifying varices and peptic ulcer disease.
- Technetium-99m-labeled RBC: scan is done with radiolabeled RBCs and can localize small active bleeds.
- Selective angiography can detect massive upper GI bleeding when other tests have failed.

Treatment
- IV fluids through a 16-gauge or larger peripheral IV, hemodynamic stability should be closely monitored.
- A Foley catheter should be inserted to assess fluid status.
- Blood products, vitamin K and antacids should be given as a prophylactic measure if the source of the bleeding remains undetermined.
- Propanolol decreases cardiac output and heart rate.
- Nitoglycerin decreases mesenteric blood flow.
- Nasogastric suction with water lavage determines if the bleeding has stopped.
- Approximately 80-85% of upper GI-bleeds will stop bleeding spontaneously.
- If the source of bleeding cannot be identified or if there is hemodynamic instability, patients should be taken to the OR.
- Once the source of bleeding has been identified a few techniques can be used to stop the bleeding
    - Electrocoagulation with cautery
    - Direct injection of vasoconstrictors
    - Heat probe
- Surgical management for varices includes a transjugular intrahepatic portosystem shunt:
    - Shunt from portal vein into vana cava bypasses the liver.

Lower GI-Bleeding

Common Causes of Lower GI-bleed
- Hemorrhoids are the most common cause of lower GI-bleeds.
- Diverticulosis
    - Rare before age 40.
    - Diverticula usually bleed profusely and then stop, not requiring surgery.
    - More frequent on left, bleed more on right.

- Vascular ectasia (acquired defect of veins and capillaries of the GI tract often with coexisting aortic stenosis)
    - The risk of bleeding from angiodysplasia increases with age.
    - The right colon is the most common site involved.
- Colon cancer
- Polyps
- Ischemic/infectious colitis
- IBD

Clinical Manifestations
- Pallor
- Diaphoresis
- Confusion
- Melena
- Hematochezia
- Acute blood loss may present with the following signs and symtoms:
    - Tachycardia
    - Narrow pulse pressure
    - Postural hypotension
    - Systolic hypotension
    - Syncope

Diagnosis
- Once NG-tube suction is negative suggesting a lower GI-bleeding source, anoscopy and rigid sigmoidoscoy should be performed.
- Angiography is recommended for severe bleeding.
- Colonoscopy is less valuable if the bleeding is active and severe. This is not the case for most lower GI-bleeds, which makes colonoscopy a valuable test.

Treatment
- Vasopressin is usually used as a temporary measure to resuscitate the patient and proceed with further management.
- Embolization may also stop acute bleeding but should be reserved for patients who are poor surgical candidates because it carries a 15% complication rate.
- If a patient requires more than two thirds of their circulating blood in less than 24 hours or if there is hemodynamic instability, laparotomy is indicated to identify the source of bleeding.

Hernias

General

Abdominal Anatomy
Layers of the abdominal wall
- *Skin*
    - Cutaneous nerves of the anterior abdominal wall are supplied by T7-L1.
- *Superficial fascia*
    - The superficial fascia is composed of two fatty layers:
        - A superficial layer called Camper's fascia
        - A deeper layer called Scarpa's fascia
- *External oblique muscle*
    - It is the outermost abdominal muscle. Its fibers run downwards as the muscle originates from the lower six ribs. Its aponeurisis forms the following structures:
        - **The inguinal ligament** as the aponeurosis rolls onto itself
        - **The lacunar ligament** as the fibers of the inguinal ligament rotate medially to attach onto the Cooper's ligament.
        - **The superficial inguinal ring** is formed as the aponeurosis of the muscle insert onto the pubic tubercle
- *Internal oblique muscle*
    - The fibers of the internal oblique muscle are directed obliquely upwards
- *Transversus abdominis muscle*
    - It is the deepest of the abdominal wall muscles and its fibers run transversely. The aponeurosis of this muscle forms the following structures:
        - **Cooper's ligament** is formed as the aponeurosis of this muscle rolls onto itself and inserts onto the pubic tubercle
        - **The internal inguinal ring** is formed by a triangular orifice of the aponeurosis of this muscle as it inserts onto the pubis.
- *Transversalis fascia*
    - The trasversalis fascia is deep to the abdominal muscles and forms an envelope of the interior abdominal cavity.
- *Peritoneum*
    - The peritoneum is the final layer of the anterior abdominal wall. It covers all intra-abodominal structures. In the scrotum, the peritoneum continues as the tunica vaginalis of the testis.

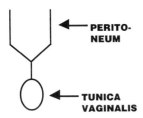

PERITO-
NEUM

TUNICA
VAGINALIS

During development there is complete obliteration of the processus vaginalis, which provides direct communication between the scrotum and the peritoneum. Failure of this process to occur may result in the formation of hydrocoeles and is a predisposing factor in the formation of indirect inguinal hernias.

• Most of the abdominal layers continue as layers in the scrotum:

Anterior abdominal wall	Scrotum
1. Peritoneum	Tunica vaginalis
2. Transversalis fascia	Internal spermatic fascia
3. Internal oblique	Cremaster
4. External oblique aponeurosis	External spermatic fascia
5. Subcutaneus fat	Colles' fascia
6. Skin	Skin

COVERINGS OF THE SPERMATIC CORD (DUCTUS DEFERENS, TESTICULAR ARTERY, VENUS PLEXUS)

Types of Hernias
• An abdominal hernia is a protrusion of any organ (or portion of it) or a structure through an abdominal defect, which may be congenital, acquired or iatrogenic.

Inguinal Hernias

* • *Indirect inguinal hernia*
  - It is a hernia that protrudes through the internal inguinal ring.
  - It contains a sac (processus vaginalis and peritoneum).
  - It is a congenital hernia. Patency of the processus vaginalis is required but not sufficient for its formation.
  - Groin hernias occurs most commonly on the right.
  - This is the most common type of hernia in both men and women.
  - This is the most common type of hernia in young patients.
  - Indirect inguinal hernias occur lateral to the inferior epigastric vessels.

- *Direct inguinal hernia*
  - ✗- Direct inguinal hernia protrudes through Hesselbach's triangle and medial to the inferior epigastric vessels.
  - - Direct inguinal hernias are usually the result of abdominal wall weakening and occur most often in older individuals. Thus, this is an acquired type of hernia.

- *Femoral Hernia*
  - - A femoral hernia protrudes through the femoral ring, which is limited medially by the **lacunar ligament**, posteriorly by **Cooper's ligament** and anteriorly by the **inguinal ligament**.
  - - This is usually an acquired lesion, which results from muscular weakening.
  - A femoral hernia is the type of hernia most susceptible to incarceration.

> - **Incarceration** refers to the entrapment of abdominal organs or part of the organ within the hernial defect. It is a hernia that does not reduce.
>
> - **Strangulation** refers to severe entrapment of an abdominal organ or part of it leading to blood supply compromise and subsequent necrosis of the entrapped organ.

Common types of hernias

Hernia type	Male	Female	Children
Direct	40%	Rare	Rare
Indirect	50%	70%	100%
Femoral	10%	30%	Rare

Other types of abdominal hernias

- **Pantaloon hernia** is a combination of both direct and indirect herniation.
- **Incisional hernia** is a hernia through an incisional site. It usually occurs as a result of incomplete closure of previous abdominal surgery. There may also be subsequent development of an infection at this site.
- **Petit's hernia** is a hernia that protrudes through the inferior lumbar triangle (lateral margin of latissimus dorsi, the medial margin of the external oblique, and the iliac crest). This type of hernia is not common.
- **Grynfeltt's hernia** is a hernia that protrudes through the superior lumbar triangle (sacrospinalis muscle, internal oblique muscle, and the inferior margin

of the 12th rib). This type of hernia is rare.

- **Spigelian hernia** is a hernia through the linea semilunaris.
- **Richter's hernia** is an incarcerated or strangulated hernia involving one side of the bowel wall. Because the lumen of the bowel is still patent, bowel necrosis may occur in the absence of bowel obstruction.
- **Littré's hernia** is any groin hernia that involves Meckel's diverticulum. These are usually incarcerated or strangulated hernias.
- **Obturator hernia** occurs as protrusion of abdominal structures pass through the obturator canal. These are much more common in females and most present as Richter's hernias.

Clinical presentation

- Most hernias present as an intermittent mass in the groin.
- There is occasional discomfort and pain with the mass.
- It is often possible to reproduce the symptoms of a hernia by voluntarily increasing of abdominal pressure as in the Valsalva maneuver or by coughing.
- In some hernias the only presenting symptoms may be those of bowel obstruction.

Diagnosis

- The diagnosis of a hernia is primarily made by physical examination.
- During physical examination, reduction of a hernia must be evaluated.

Treatment

- In older patients with large hernias, the risk of strangulation is remote. In this case elective surgical repair must be carefully considered by assessing the risk of surgery versus the risk of incarceration.
- The natural history of hernias is to incarcerate and strangulate. A reducible hernia is an elective procedure. Incarcerated hernias are surgical emergencies.
  - Inguinal hernias: 3% incarcerate in the first three months.
  - Femoral hernias: 20% incarcerate in the first three months.

The Esophagus

- The following are disorders of the esophagus:

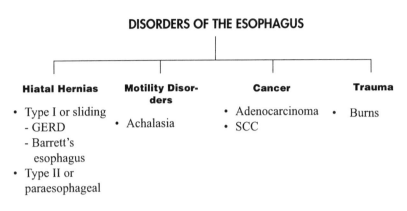

DISORDERS OF THE ESOPHAGUS

Hiatal Hernias	Motility Disorders	Cancer	Trauma

• Type I or sliding
  - GERD
  - Barrett's
    esophagus
• Type II or
  paraesophageal
	• Achalasia	• Adenocarcinoma
		• SCC
			• Burns

Hiatal Hernia

- Hiatal hernias occur as a result of a defect of the phrenoesophageal membrane.

- **Type I** or sliding hernia is characterized by laxity at the gastroesophageal hiatus allowing the distal esophagus and gastric cardia to herniate through it.

  - The diagnosis is made by esophagoscopy and is established when at least two cm of gastric mucosa is seen between the hiatus of the diaphragm and the gastroesophageal junction.

- **Type II** or paraesophageal hernia is present when there is a defect in the phrenoesophageal membrane.

- The ratio of type I to type II hiatal hernias is about 100:1.

- Eighty percent of patients with sliding hernias also present with gastroesophageal reflux disease (**GERD**), a separate entity.

- **Type III** hiatal hernia is a combination of type I and type II hiatal hernias and is more common than the incidence of a pure Type II hiatal hernia.

- Risk factors for the development of hiatal hernias are associated with **increased abdominal pressure** such as **obesity** and **pregnancy**.

- **Type IV** hiatal hernia is present when abdominal contents other than, or in addition to, the stomach herniate through the paraesophageal hiatus, requiring immediate surgical intervention.

> Sliding and paraesophageal
> hernias are the most common types
> of hiatal hernias.

The following table differentiates between type I and type II hiatal hernias.

Hiatal Hernia	Clinical Presentation	Diagnosis	Treatment
Type I	• 20% are asymptomatic • 80% present with GERD (burning, nonradiating, position-dependent epigastric pain, substernal tightness) • Symptoms may be exacerbated by gastric irritants (alcohol, tobacco, caffeine) • Feeling of food stuck beneath the esophagus	• H & P does not help in diagnosis • CXR • Barium swallow • Esophageal manometric testing (establishes pressure differences) • Esophageal pH testing • Endoscopy +/- biopsy	• *Medical* (2/3 of patients respond to medical treatment) • Avoid gastric irritants (alcohol, tobacco, and caffeine). • No food intake several hours before bed. • Weight reduction • Sleep with head at 30° • Regular use of antacids • *Surgical* • Surgery should correct the anatomical defect and prevent reflux • Types of surgery include Nissen, Belsey, and Hill operations
Type II	• Usually asymptomatic. Surgery indicated without symptoms because incarceration and strangulation may occur. • Incarcerated hernias may become ischemic. Symptoms in such situations include dysphagia, bleeding, and breathlessness.	• History is contributory if symptoms develop, which suggests ischemia. • CXR (air fluid levels in the posterior mediastinum) • Barium swallow may demonstrate reflux or anatomical abnormalities.	• Type II, III, and IV hiatal hernias should be repaired surgically. • 30% of untreated hernias lead to catastrophic events • Surgical approach can be thoracic or esophageal and consists of reduction of the hernia, resection of the sac and closure of the hiatal defect.

Reflux eosphagitis

• Reflux esophagitis can occur in the absence of hiatal hernias. The pathogenesis of reflux esophagitis is unclear, but it is thought to be **multifactorial**.

• The following factors may contribute to reflux esophagitis:

  - Weakness of the lower esophageal sphincter alone has failed to reproduce the symptoms of reflux but in combination with other abnormalities may reproduce the symptoms.

  - Direct injection of acid into the esophagus reproduces the symptoms of heartburn (Bernstein test). This does not happen in the normal esophagus as the healthy esophagus can resolve the lower pH with less than ten swallows.

  - More reflux usually occurs in patients whose **intra-abdominal esophagus is short**.

  - Increased positive abdominal pressure and/or increased negative thoracic pressure may contribute to the development of symptoms.

  - The disease is caused by the duration of exposure to acid to the esophagus rather than the amount of acid present.

Complications of reflux esophagitis

• Complications include mucosal erosion, ulceration, stricture, and aspiration pneumonia.

• Chronic gastroesophageal reflux may result in **Barrett's esophagus**, which occurs when the epithelium of the distal esophagus undergoes metaplasia to resemble gastric cardiac epithelium.

  - The risk of developing **adenocarcinoma** in patients with Barrett's esophagus is 50-100 times higher than the normal population.

  - Treatment of Barrett's esophagus consists of treatment of reflux, which does not reverse the metaplastic changes but prevents its progression.

• Clinical presentation, diagnosis and treatment for reflux esophagitis are indicated in the table above. Medical treatment is the major form of management of reflux esophagitis.

• If medical management fails, surgery is indicated.

  - The transabdominal approach is preferred over transthoracic because of lower morbidity.

  - Surgical mortality is less than one percent.

  - Postoperative complications include dysphagia, inability to vomit and splenic injury.

  - Repair is done with a Nissen fundoplication, which is usually done laparoscopically.

Esophageal Motility Disorders

Achalasia

General

* Achalasia is the most common motility disorder of the esophagus. It is a disorder in which the lower esophageal sphincter (**LES**) fails to relax during swallowing.

Clinical presentation
* Dysphagia
* Regurgitation of undigested solid and liquid food
* Weight loss
* Aspiration pneumonia
* May lead to the formation of diverticula
    - Diverticula are outpouchings of part or the entire esophagus. Treatment consists of excision of the diverticula and treatment of the underlying disease. Cervical diverticula are called Zenker's diverticula.

Diagnosis
* Radiographic contrast studies classically reveal dilatation of the esophagus.
* Manometry studies reveal increased pressure of the LES.
* Endoscopy should be performed with caution because diverticula can be perforated.

Treatment
* Myotomy of the LES is the mainstay of treatment.
* Balloon dilatation of the LES is an alternative in poor candidates for surgery.

Esophageal Cancer

General
* Common malignant lesions of the esophagus include adenocarcinoma and squamous cell carcinoma (**SSC**).
* SCC is the most common malignancy affecting the esophagus, usually the proximal part.
* Adenocarcinoma usually occurs in the distal esophagus.

Risk Factors for Adenocarcinoma
* White race

- Gastroesophageal reflux and Barrett's esophagus (10%)

Risk Factors for SCC

- Black race
- Alcohol and tobacco use
- Achalasia or diverticula of the esophagus
- Diet or vitamin deficiency
- Poor oral hygiene

Clinical Presentation

- Dysphagia
- Weight loss
- Pain
- When pain is present, it is a severe substernal pain with fever and tachycardia.
- The symptoms of esophageal cancer are usually insidious and occur only after the disease has progressed significantly, resulting in poor prognosis.

Diagnosis

- Barium swallow should be the first study done to establish the diagnosis.
- The diagnosis is usually confirmed by endoscopy and biopsy.
- Evaluation of lymph nodes and distal metastasis is usually done with CT scan.

Treatment

- Surgical resection is the mainstay of treatment.
- Chemotherapy may improve the 5-year survival rate, but the overall cure rate for esophageal cancer is only about five pecent.
- Surgery versus chemotherapy and radiation therapy are approximately as effective treatments for SCC.

Esophageal Trauma

General

- Perforation of the esophagus occurs frequently in trauma patients.
- Perforation can occur intraluminally or extraluminally.

Intraluminal	Extraluminal
· Instrumental injuries represent about 75% of esophageal injuries (NG tube passage) · Foreign body · Cancer	· Penetrating injuries · Blunt trauma · Operative injury

> **Boerhaave's syndrome** is a form of esophageal perforation that occurs following emesis and involves all layers of the esophagus. The syndrome occurs frequently in alcoholics following emesis against a closed epiglottis.

Clinical presentation of esophageal perforation

- Dysphagia
- Chest or abdominal pain
- Diaphoresis
- Leukocytosis
- Tachycardia
- Respiratory distress

Diagnosis

- History and physical
- CXR
- Barium swallow
- Endoscopy

Treatment

- NPO
- NG-tube suctioning
- IV hydration
- Broad spectrum antibiotics
- Emergent surgical repair of the esophageal perforation

- Early perforation is surgically repaired by primary repair.

- Late perforation is surgically repaired by diversion of the esophagus (cervical esophagostomy), stapling of the stomach and draining of the mediastinum—There is very high mortality in patients with late perforation.

The Stomach

Physiology of Acid Secretion

There are three phases of hydrochloric acid secretion:

* **Cephalic**, which is mediated by the vagus nerve's release of ACh.
* **Gastric**, which is mediated by the antral release of gastrin.
* **Intestinal**, which is mediated by the small intestine's release of peptides and histamine.

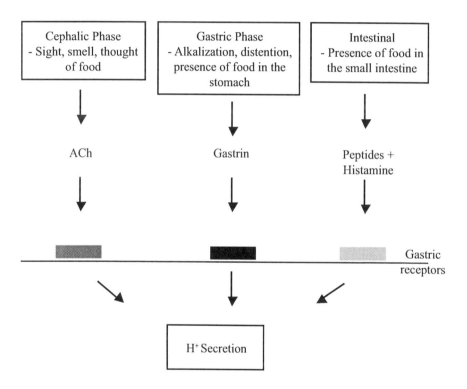

Peptic Ulcer Disease

General

* Peptic ulcer disease (**PUD**) occurs when the defense mechanisms of the gastrointestinal tract are unable to deal with acid secretion, which results in autodigestion of the mucosa.

* Peptic ulcer disease refers to both **gastric** and **duodenal ulcers**. These ulcers have different characteristics.

Duodenal Ulcers

General

- Duodenal ulcers occur as a result of excessive acid secretion.
- These are twice as common as gastric ulcers.
- Duodenal ulcer perforate more frequently than gastric ulcers.
- They occur more commonly in men than women.
- They occur most frequently in the 40-60-year-old patient population.

Clinical Presentation

- The clinical presentation of duodenal ulcers depends on the severity and duration of the ulcers as well as the presence of complications.
- The following complications are observed in duodenal ulcers:
    - Intractability
    - Hemorrhage
    - Obstruction
    - Perforation
- Epigastric pain that is exacerbated by fasting and ameliorated by antacids and food is a classic presentation of duodenal ulcers.
- Bleeding may result if **perforation** has occurred.
    - The bleeding may be massive if erosion into the gastroduodenal artery has occurred.
    - Symptoms suggestive of bleeding are primarily hemodynamic ($\downarrow$BP, $\uparrow$ HR, syncope).
- Perforation may also produce the signs and symptoms of an acute abdomen.
- X-ray may reveal the presence of free air.

Diagnosis

- History and physical examination. An important element in the history is drastic changes in food habits and epigastric pain.
- Upper GI series consisting of barium swallows.
- Endoscopy is even more accurate than upper GI series.
- Gastric acid analysis consists of NG-tube placement in the stomach and acid collection every 15 minutes for two hours. After an hour, histamine antagonists are given and the basal rate for cephalic acid secretion is assessed. Patients with PUD usually have high basal acid output. However, this test is rarely done.

Gastrointestinal Bleeding

General

- Peptic ulcer disease (**PUD**) occurs when the defense mechanisms of the gastrointestinal tract are unable to deal with acid secretion, which results in autodigestion of the mucosa.
- Peptic ulcer disease refers to both **gastric** and **duodenal ulcers**. These ulcers have different characteristics.

Treatment

Medical treatment
- Decrease secretagogues and irritants
    - caffeine
    - tobacco use
    - alcohol
    - chocolate
    - peppermint
- Intraluminal antacids
- Histamine blockers
    - cimetidine
    - famotidine
- Anticholinergics
- H^+ pump inhibitors
    - omeprazole
    - lansoprazole
- *H. pylori* **eradication** with any of a number of antibiotic regimens.
    - bismuth subsalicylate, metronidazole, and tetracycline for two weeks.

Surgical treatment
- Surgical treatment is indicated if duodenal ulcer is complicated by Intractability, Obstruction, Hemorrhage, or Perforation.
    - Assessment of ABCs should be the first step in the management of ulcer complications.
    - Patients with a suspected perforation or a patient requiring more than six units of blood in 24 h should undergo exploratory laparotomy.

Common operations for PUD
- As the cephalic phase of acid secretion is usually the culprit in PUD, the aim of surgical intervention is to interrupt the vagal stimulation of acid secretion.
- This can be accomplished in one of three ways:

1. Truncal vagotomy
2. Selective vagotomy
3. Proximal gastric vagotomy

1. Truncal Vagotomy

    *   Truncal vagotomy is a complete transection of the vagus nerve just above the esophageal hiatus of the diaphragm. This procedure denervates:
        -   Parietal cells
        -   Antral pump mechanisms
        -   Pyloric sphincter mechanisms
        -   Abdominal viscera
    *   As this procedure disrupts pumping mechanisms, a second operation usually accompanies truncal vagotomy to restore stomach emptying. This is often called "a drainage procedure".
        -   **Pyloroplasty** is a drainage procedure that consists of a horizontal incision of the pylorus, which is subsequently repaired vertically.
    *   Operations done for reconstruction following antrectomy include:
        -   **Billroth I operation** consists of anterectomy with gastroduodenostomy.
        -   **Billroth II operation** consists of an anterectomy with gastrojejunostomy.
        -   **Roux-en-Y operation**
            -   A jejunostomy is performed forming a Y-shaped figure of small bowel followed by a gastrojejunostomy.
    *   As performing an anterectomy augments the effects of the vagotomy by eliminating the gastric phase of acid secretion together with the cephalic phase, anterectomy with truncal vagotomy has the **lowest recurrence rate of PUD**. However, it also has the **highest rate of postgastrectomy syndromes**.

2. Selective Vagotomy

    *   Selective vagotomy provides a total denervation of the stomach from the crus of the diaphragm down and including the pylorus.
    *   This procedure spares the parasympathetic innervation to the abdominal viscera but also interferes with gastric motility requiring a drainage procedure (pyloroplasty).
    *   The rate of postgastrectomy syndromes with this procedure is the same as truncal vagotomy.

3. Proximal Gastric Vagotomy

    *   In this procedure, only the branches of the nerves that supply the parietal cells are divided.
    *   Pyloric sphincter and antral pumping mechanisms are spared and a drainage procedure is not required. Thus, this procedure has the **lowest rate of postgastric syndromes**. However, the **highest incidence of PUD recurrence** is observed with this procedure.

Gastric Ulcers

General

- The etiology of gastric ulcers is unclear. The hydrochloric acid load is typically normal to mildly elevated.

- Possible mechanisms include:
  - defective mucosal barrier
  - delayed gastric emptying
  - history of gastritis

- Gastric ulcers usually occur in the lesser curvature.

- Gastric ulcers have a higher rate of bleeding but lower rate of perforation.

- In contrast to duodenal ulcers, **gastric ulcers may be associated** with malignancy.

Clinical presentation

- In contrast to duodenal ulcers, the pain of gastric ulcers occurs in the epigastrium and is exacerbated by the ingestion of food.

- Weight loss is also a common presentation of gastric ulcers.

Diagnosis

- Upper GI series

- Endoscopy: because of the associated risk of malignancy with gastric ulcer, multiple biopsies should be taken during endoscopy.

Treatment

Medical treatment

- A smaller percentage of gastric ulcers respond to medical treatment compared to duodenal ulcers.

- The medical management of gastric ulcers is essentially the same as for duodenal ulcers with the exception of anticholinergic drug therapy as these are contraindicated in gastric ulcers.

- Prostaglandin blocking medications should be stopped.
  - aspirin
  - NSAIDs
  - steroids

Surgical treatment

- Distal gastrectomy with excision of the ulcer is generally successful in the majority of cases and has a very small recurrence rate.

Zollinger-Ellison Syndrome

General
- This syndrome is caused by the direct production of gastrin by a tumor usually arising in the pancreas or paraduodenal area.
- About two thirds of these tumors are malignant.

Clinical presentation
- Patients usually present with intractable duodenal ulcers

Diagnosis
- The diagnosis is made by gastrin serum levels above 300 pg/ ml. However, this is not always seen. The diagnosis can be confirmed with secreting stimulation test.

Treatment
- Medical treatment consists of histamine blockers and H^+ pump blockers.
- Surgery is performed if an isolated identifiable tumor is localized.
    - If the tumor is not localized, proximal gastric vagotomy in combination with medical treatment is indicted.
    - Definitive treatment consists of total gastrectomy as this entirely eliminates the source of acid. This is rarely performed.

Gastric cancer

General
- The incidence of gastric cancer in the United States is low compared to Japan, China, and Finland.
- Environmental and dietary factors have been advocated as possible etiologic agents.
- Most gastric carcinomas originate in the distal half of the stomach, in the pyloric gland area.
- Risk factors for the development of gastric cancer include:
    - Adenomatous polyps
    - Chronic gastritis
    - Achlorhydria
    - Gastic ulcer disease

Clinical manifestations
* The signs and symptoms of gastric cancer usually present late when the disease is far advanced. The symptoms include:
    - Weight loss
    - Epigastric pain
    - Hematemesis
    - Dysphagia
    - Melena
    - Metastatic disease occurs to:
        - regional lymph nodes
        - the left supraclavicular area (Virchow's node)
        - omentum
        - ovary (Krukenberg's tumors)
        - umbilicus (Sister Joseph's nodule)
    - Obstruction

Diagnosis
* Upper GI series
* Endoscopy with biopsy

Treatment
* Complete surgical resection of the stomach
    - Extended surgical resection removes the spleen, distal pancreas, parapyloric nodes and omentum.
* The 5-year survival rate depends on the stage of the cancer.
* Due to the late diagnosis of gastric carcinoma, the 5-year survival rate in the United States is about 10%.

STAGING OF GASTRIC CANCER

Stage I	Stage II	Stage III	Stage IV
• Invasion through the muscularis mucosae • (-) nodes	• Invasion through the muscularis externa • (-) nodes	• Invasion through the muscularis externa • (+) nodes	• (+) nodes • distal metastasis

The Small Intestine

Small Bowel Obstruction (SBO)

General
- Mechanical obstruction of the small bowel is a common cause of acute abdomen in the surgical patient.
- In SBO, there is mechanical obstruction to the passage of intraluminal contents, which gives rise to the signs and symptoms observed.

Clinical Presentation
- Nausea and vomiting
- Intermittent crampy abdominal pain
- Abdominal distension
- High-pitched bowel sounds
- **Constipation**
- **Obstipation** (inability to pass flatus, which occurs in complete bowel obstruction)
- Fluid and electrolyte imbalances
    - This occurs secondary to large amounts of isotonic fluid loss into the intestinal lumen.
    - Up to eight liters of fluid can be sequestered in the lumen of the small bowel.
    - This usually leads to **hypokalemic metabolic alkalosis**
- If perforation is present, patients may present with signs and symptoms of **peritonitis** and **sepsis**.

Diagnosis
- History and physical examination
    - History of previous surgeries or cancer are important elements of history taking as surgery and cancer have a high rate of occurrence of adhesions.
    - Physical examination should investigate the presence of hernias.
    - History and physical examination is essential in differentiating between paralytic ileus and SBO (see table below).
- Acute Abdominal Series (upright chest, supine abdomen-KUB, upright abdomen)
    - The Acute Abdominal Series (AAS) films are the most useful studies to

	SBO	Paralytic Ileus	Large Bowel Obstruction
Common Causes	• Adhesions (60%) • Hernia (20%) • Tumors (15%) • Intussusception • Crohn's Disease (5%)	• Acute pancreatitis • Appendicitis • Cholecystitis • Gastroenteritis	• Colon cancer • Diverticulitis • Volvulus
History and Physical Exam	• Crampy abdominal pain • Nausea and vomiting • Constipation and obstipation • High pitched bowel sounds or absent in complete obstruction	• Minimal continuos abdominal pain • Nausea and vomiting • Constipation and obstipation • Absent bowel sounds	• Crampy abdominal pain • Nausea and vomiting • Constipation and obstipation • High pitched or absent bowel sounds
AAS Findings	• Dilated loops of small bowel occupying the center of the abdomen • Small, closely spaced mucosal folds • Little or no colonic gas • Differential air fluid levels	• In prone position, air will flow to rectum if no obstruction. Thus, there are large amounts of gas in the small intestine and colon	• Dilated loops of bowel occupying the periphery of the abdomen • Widely spaced haustrations • Gas in the rectum and dilated colon

establish the diagnosis and distinguish SBO from paralytic ileus and large bowel obstruction, all of which usually produce similar signs and symptoms.

• Plain films should also be used to exclude SBO complications such as perforation, which may be manifested by the presence of free air on upright films.

• Barium enema is also used in the diagnosis of SBO if there is still uncertainty with the AAS studies.

• Laboratory tests (electrolytes, BUN, creatinine, CBC) should be obtained to assess the fluid and electrolyte status and infection.

Treatment

- ABCs should be assessed first. Patients with severe dehydration should be appropriately resuscitated.
- Patients with complete bowel obstruction should undergo exploratory laparotomy since a major risk with SBO is the development of strangulation.
- The goals of the operation are to relieve the obstruction (by e.g., lysis of adhesions (LOA), hernia repair, untwisting of volvulus) and to resect any necrotic bowel.
- Partial obstruction can be managed with a trial of NG decompression.

Malignant Neoplasms of the Small Bowel

- The most common cancers of the small bowel include (in order of frequency):
  - Adenocarcinoma
    - 1% of GI malignancies
    - This is the most common malignancy of the small bowel.
    - Order of occurrence is usually duodenum >ileum >jejunum.
  - Carcinoid tumors
    - These are cancers that originate from a neuroectodermal origin; thus, also known as APUDomas (amine precursor uptake and decarboxylation).
    - They have high potential for metastasis and are considered malignant.
    - The small bowel is the second most common location (ileum > jejunum) for these tumors. More than 50% of carcinoid tumors occur in the appendix.
    - They produce large amounts of serotonin
  - Lymphoma
    - It represents the most common malignancy of the small bowel in the pediatric population.
    - It commonly occurs in the ileum.
  - Leiomyosarcomas

Clinical manifestations

- Adenocarcinoma
  - Usually causes intermittent or partial SBO
- Carcinoids
  - May present as the carcinoid syndrome:
    - Cutaneus flushing
    - Bronchospasm and wheezing
    - Valvular heart diseaseà right sided heart failure
    - Chronic watery diarrhea
- Lymphoma
  - Anorexia and weight loss

- Anemia
- SBO

Diagnosis

1. Adenocarcinoma
   - Stool occult blood
   - Barium contrast x-rays
   - Fiber optic endoscopy
2. Carcinoids
   - Elevated serum serotonin
   - Elevated 5-HIAA in the urine

Treatment

1. Adenocarcinoma
   - Wide surgical excision of the tumor including mesenteric lymph nodes
   - There is a 20-30% five year survival due to late diagnosis.
2. Carcinoids
   - Medical
     - Octeotride infusion
     - Chemotherapy
   - Surgical
     - Surgical resection, although excision of the tumor does not seem to affect survival rate
3. Lymphoma
   - Wide surgical excision including mesenteric lymph nodes

Colon

Diverticular Disease

General

- **Diverticula** are sacs or pouches of tubular or vesicular organs. They may occur in any segment along the GI tract. Diverticular disease typically refers to the presence of diverticula in the colon. There are two types of diverticula: true diverticula and false diveticula.

    - *True Diverticula* are pouches in the bowel wall involving all of its layers. These types of diverticula are not common in the colon and are usually congenital. Right sided diverticula of the colon are more common in young patients.

    - *False diverticula* are pouches of the bowel wall involving only the mucosal and submucosal layers. These diverticula are the most common type encountered in the colon and > 90% occur in the sigmoid colon.

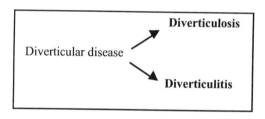

- **Diverticulosis** is the presence of one or more diverticula in the colon.
- **Diverticulitits** occurs when infection is present in one or more diverticula.

Diverticulosis

Clinical Manifestations

- The majority of patients with uncomplicated diverticulosis are asymptomatic.

- A small fraction of patients with uncomplicated diverticulosis may complain of left lower quadrant abdominal pain and changes in bowel habits such as constipation or diarrhea.

- Patients presenting with bright red blood per rectum (BRBPR) are at risk of massive bleeding (those patients requiring > 6 U of blood in < 24 h) if it is due to diverticulosis. The clinical presentation and management of diverticular bleeding is outlined in the lower GI bleed section.

- Complications of diverticulosis:
    - 20% of patients develop diverticulitis
    - 5-10% of patients suffer from diverticular bleeding

Diagnosis

- The diagnosis of uncomplicated diverticulosis is difficult to make in the absence of symptoms.

- When diverticulosis is complicated by diverticulitis or diverticular bleeding a workup consisting of barium enema and colonoscopy is indicated. This should be done at least six weeks after the acute phase.

Management

- The management of uncomplicated diverticulosis is non-operative and consists of a high-fiber diet.

- The management of diverticular bleeding is outlined in the lower GI bleed section.

Diverticulitis

Clinical Manifestations

Uncomplicated Diverticulitis:

- Left lower quadrant abdominal pain

- Constipation/diarrhea

- Fever/leukocytosis

- Complications of diverticulitis and clinical presentation:
  - Perforations (45%)
    - Clinical presentation varies from spontaneous resolution to the presence of an acute abdomen.
  - Abscess (10%)
    - Fever
    - Leukocytosis
    - Localized abdominal tenderness
    - Acute abdomen
  - Obstruction (5%)
    - Abdominal distension
    - Nausea and vomiting
    - Constipation/obstipation
    - Abdominal tenderness
  - Fistula formation (4%)
    - Colovesical fistula (most common type); UTI is the most common presentation
    - Colovaginal fistula
    - Colocutanesus fistula

Diagnosis

- The diagnosis is made primarily by history and physical examination.
- Barium enema and colonoscopy should not be done in the acute phase of the clinical complication as perforation may occur during these procedures.
- AAS may reveal signs of free air (suggesting perforation) or dilated loops and air fluid levels (suggesting obstruction).
- CT-scan is most useful and can be performed in the acute phase.

Management

- Mild diverticulitis:
    - May be treated with oral antibiotics in some instances
- Moderate to severe diverticulitis:
    - ABCs
    - NPO
    - IV antibiotics
- Complications:
    - Free perforation
        - Exploratory laparotomy
        - Sigmoid colectomy with end colostomy (Hartmann's procedure)
    - Abscess
        - CT-scan guided drainage or OR drainage
        - Obstruction
        - Sigmoid resection with colostomy (Hartmann's procedure)

Colonic Polyps

General
- A polyp is a mucosal and/or submucosal growth into the lumen of the bowel.
- Premalignant polyps are adenomas.
- These polyps can be sessile (flat and closely attached to the mucosal surface) or pedunculated (round and attached to the mucosal surface by a thin neck).
- The polyp can be tubular (rod-like), villous (finger-like), or a combination of both (tubulovillous).

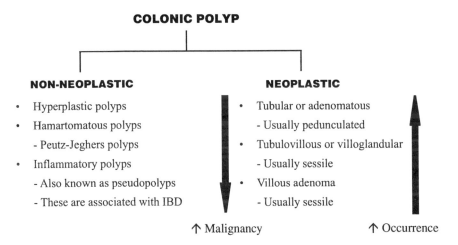

COLONIC POLYP

NON-NEOPLASTIC
- Hyperplastic polyps
- Hamartomatous polyps
  - Peutz-Jeghers polyps
- Inflammatory polyps
  - Also known as pseudopolyps
  - These are associated with IBD

↑ Malignancy

NEOPLASTIC
- Tubular or adenomatous
  - Usually pedunculated
- Tubulovillous or villoglandular
  - Usually sessile
- Villous adenoma
  - Usually sessile

↑ Occurrence

Clinical Manifestations
- Polyps that have not progressed into carcinoma are usually asymptomatic.
- Some polyps may present with bleeding and change in bowel habits (diarrhea/constipation).

Diagnosis
- The presence of polyps is usually established as a result of screening for another condition such as colon cancer or inflammatory bowel disease (IBD) by barium enema or colonoscopy.
- About 5% of all barium enemas performed reveal the presence of polyps in the asymptomatic patient.

Management
- Once the presence of polyps has been established, removal by colonoscopy is indicated.
- Histologic evaluation should be performed to exclude the possibility of cancer.

- If a polyp is found to be adenomatous, a **full colonoscopy** (i.e. to cecum) should be performed to exclude the presence of any other polyps in the rest of the colon.

Polyposis Syndromes

1. **Familial adenomatous polyposis coli (FAP)** is an autosomal dominant disease with 100% penetrance in which affected individuals develop hundreds of adenomatous polyps in the colon and rectum beginning early in adolescence. Patients with this syndrome will inevitably develop colon cancer if untreated. FAP occurs as a result of a mutation of the Adenomatous Polyposis Coli (APC) gene. APC is lost early in sporadic colon cancer in the adenoma-carcinoma sequence of colon cancer. Patients with a family history of FAP should be under close surveillance for the development of polyps. Patients found to have polyps should undergo prophylactic colectomy.

2. **Gardner's syndrome** is a variant of FAP in which in addition to the hundreds of adenomatous colonic and rectal polyps there are extraintestinal manifestations, such as desmoid tumors (tumors of the musculoaponeurotic sheath), osteomas (of the skull), and sebaceous cysts. Gardner's syndrome is also an autosomal dominant disease, but it has a variable degree of penetrance.

3. **Turcot's syndrome** is a variant of FAP consisting of colonic polyps and CNS malignancy (gliomas).

4. **Peutz-Jeghers syndrome** is a syndrome characterized by hamartomatous polyps throughout the GI tract with the following order of incidence: jejunum > ileum > colon > stomach. Patients with this syndrome present with mucocutaneous pigmentation. Extraintestinal malignancy of the ovaries, breast and thyroid are also associated with this syndrome.

Colon Cancer

General

- Colorectal carcinoma is the fourth most common cancer and the second leading cause of death due to cancer in the United States.
- Most deaths occur because colorectal cancer is usually diagnosed symptomatically when the disease has advanced to an aggressive stage.
- In 5% of the cases, colon cancer occurs together with rectal cancer (synchronous) and in 5% of the cases, colon cancer recurs after surgical resection of the first cancer.
- Distribution of colon cancer:

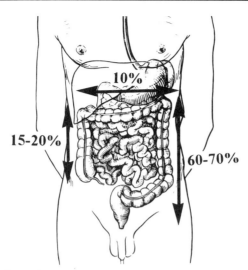

Risk Factors for colon cancer

- **Ulcerative colitis** → ↑ risk to 10% at 10 years and 1% per year thereafter.

- **1ˢᵗ degree relatives with colon cancer** due to genetic alterations of any or all of the following chromosomes 5 (APC), 12 (k-ras), 17 (p53), and18 (DCC), → ↑ risk by 10-15%.

- **Familial adenomatous polyposis (FAP)** → 5% of colon cancers are related to FAP. All patients with FAP will develop colon cancer before the age of 40 if untreated.

- **Lynch syndrome or hereditary nonpolyposis colorectal cancer (HNPCC)**→ represents 2% of bowel cancers

- **Age** → incidence ↑ significantly by age 50 and peaks at age 70. Patients > 70 years old present with an earlier stage of colon cancer and have better outcome than younger patients.

- **Environment/diet** → High fat intake and low fiber intake (Western diet).

Clinical Manifestations

- The clinical manifestations of colon cancer depend on the site that is affected:

Sign/symptom	Right colon	Left colon
1. Abdominal, pelvic or back pain	Common	Common
2. Obstruction/ perforation	Uncommon	Common
3. Weight loss	Common	Uncommon
4. Anemia	Common	Uncommon
5. Melena	Common	Uncommon
6. Hematochezia	Uncommon	Common

- Hematochezia = blood in stools
- Melena = black stools which are colored due to the presence of partly digested blood.

Diagnosis

• History and physical examination
- Family history of colon cancer and/or polyps
- History of ulcerative colitis
- Recent change in bowel habits
- Easily fatigued
- Melena/hematochezia
• Digital rectal examination (DRE)
• Hemoccult testing has been shown to reduce colon cancer mortality in patients >50 years old when performed every year.
• Flexible sigmidoscopy and BE
• Colonoscopy

Screening Guidelines for Colon Cancer

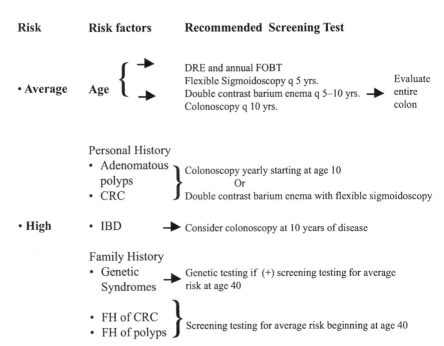

Risk	Risk factors	Recommended Screening Test
• Average	Age	DRE and annual FOBT Flexible Sigmoidoscopy q 5 yrs. Double contrast barium enema q 5–10 yrs. → Evaluate entire colon Colonoscopy q 10 yrs.
• High	Personal History • Adenomatous polyps • CRC	Colonoscopy yearly starting at age 10 Or Double contrast barium enema with flexible sigmoidoscopy
	• IBD	→ Consider colonoscopy at 10 years of disease
	Family History • Genetic Syndromes	→ Genetic testing if (+) screening testing for average risk at age 40
	• FH of CRC • FH of polyps	Screening testing for average risk beginning at age 40

Management

- Preoperative **full colonoscopy** is indicated to detect synchronous lesions. If this is not possible preoperatively due to obstruction, exploration should be performed during surgical resection of the primary tumor.

- **Carcinoembryonic antigen (CEA)** is an adhesion molecule that is overexpressed in the great majority of colon cancers. This is not a screening test but should be obtained preoperatively to determine the baseline level and assess recurrence after surgery.

- **Liver function tests (LFTs)** should be obtained as part of the preoperative laboratory tests. This may help assess possible metastasis to the liver (alkaline phosphatase is the most useful LFT). The liver is a common site of distal metastasis from colon cancer due to portal hematogenous spread. However, the **most common site of metastasis occurs to regional lymph nodes**. Workup for distal metastasis without symptoms is not recommended during the first presentation of colon cancer malignancy. Thus, CT scan is not routinely obtained for a patient initially presenting with colon cancer to evaluate for distal metastasis nor should it be obtained to attempt to stage the malignancy. While staging is an essential predictor of prognosis, staging is most accurately done by operative exploration and pathology after resection of the cancer.

Colon Cancer Treatment

- The mainstay for the treatment of colon cancer is **surgical resection**. Surgical resection includes removal of local lymph nodes and blood supply to the colon involved with at least 5-cm margins.

- Tumors involving adjacent organs should include resection of the affected organ when possible (e.g., cystectomy, hysterectomy).

- When preparation is not possible due to obstruction or perforation, a diverting colostomy (dissection of the colon where the proximal end is brought to a surgically created defect in the abdominal wall) should be performed with reanastomosis of the colon at a later date.

Rectal Cancer Treatment

- **Low anterior resection (LAR)** is performed for in all tumors in the upper one third of the rectum and some middle third tumors. It consists of resection of tumor with primary anastomosis.

- **Abdominal perineal resection (APR)** is usually recommended in some middle third tumors and all lower third of the rectum tumors. It consists of resection of rectum and a diverting colostomy.

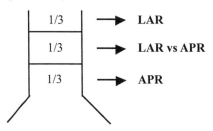

Adjuvant Therapy

- 5-fluorouracil (5-FU) and levamisole lower mortality by about 30% in patients with Dukes stage C colorectal cancer. Efficacy has not been established for other tumor stages.
- Preoperative and postoperative radiotherapy can reduce local recurrence after surgery for rectal cancer.

Prognosis

- The prognosis of colorectal cancer depends on the histological stage of the cancer.
- Traditionally the Dukes classification system has been employed. This is now being replaced by the TNM staging system.

TNM	DUKES	Description	Nodes	% 5-year survival
I (T1N0M0)	A	Confined to the mucosa	(-)	90-95
II (T2N0M0)	B1	Extension to the muscularis externa	(-)	80-85
(T3N0M0)	B2	Extension through the muscularis externa	(-)	70-75
III (T2N1M0)	C1	Extension to the muscularis externa	(+)	40-50
(T3N1M0)	C2	Extension through the muscularis externa	(+)	30-40
IV any T, any N, M1	D	Distal metastsis	(+/-)	<5

Follow-up

- Colon cancer recurrence is high. Thus, appropriate follow-up is essential.
- Regular physical examinations every three months.
- CEA level determination every three months is indicated after surgical intervention.
- Colonoscopy or barium enema should be performed every six months after surgery for the first two years.

Inflammatory Bowel Disease (IBD)

Ulcerative Colitis and Crohn's Disease

General
- Ulcerative colitis and Crohn's Disease are two disorders typically grouped together under inflammatory bowel disease (**IBD**).
- The etiology of these disorders in not understood.
- The following similarities are found in these disorders:

- **Common extraintestinal symptoms**:
  - Ankylosing spondylitis
  - Oral ulcers
  - Kidney pathology
  - Arthritis
  - Erythema nodosum
  - Clubbing of the fingers
  - Sclerosing cholangitis
- **Affected population**
  - ↑ incidence in Jewish population
  - ↓ incidence in African-American population
- **Medical treatment**
  - Sulfasalazine
  - Steroids

- Because of their similarities, these disorders are usually grouped together. However, important differences exist in each of these diseases (see table below).

Clinical Presentation

- **Ulcerative colitis (UC)**
  - Weight loss
  - Fever
  - Abdominal pain
  - **Bloody diarrhea** due to **mucosal involvement** characteristic of **UC**.

- **Crohn's disease (CD)**
  - Weight loss
  - Fever

- Diarrhea
- **Perforation**
- **Perianal fistulas** } Due to characteristic transmural involvement
- Obstruction

COMMON FISTULAS THAT OCCUR IN CD

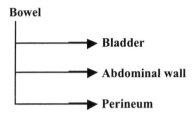

Bowel
- → **Bladder**
- → **Abdominal wall**
- → **Perineum**

- Bowel to bladder fistulas are the most common and present with UTIs.

Diagnosis
- History and physical examination
    - Important signs are bloody diarrhea for UC and obstruction/fistula formation for CD
- Colonoscopy
- Barium enema

The following are differences in these disorders which are important in the diagnosis:

	Ulcerative Colitis	**Crohn's Disease**
GI Distribution	Limited to the colon	Involves entire GI tract
Pattern along GI tract	Continuous	Intermittent with skipped lesions
Bowel wall involvement	Limited to the mucosa	Entire bowel wall
Colon cancer risk	High	Low

Management
- Medical management
  - **Sulfasalazine** is taken up by affected tissue and then converted to aminosalicylate, which is anti-inflammatory.
  - **Steroids** have many significant side effects and should only be used in acute flare-ups and tapered soon after resolution of the acute flare-up.
- In UC there are more acute flare-ups with remission. Episodes of CD are more indolent and chronic. UC responds to medical treatment better than CD.
- **Surgical intervention** is indicated when medical treatment fails or complications occur. Surgical intervention in **UC** is usually performed due to intractability of the disease in which case surgery is **therapeutic. Surgery for CD is usually palliative.**
- Complications of IBD

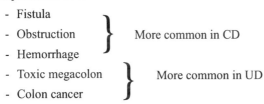

  - Fistula
  - Obstruction   } More common in CD
  - Hemorrhage
  - Toxic megacolon   } More common in UD
  - Colon cancer

Toxic Megacolon
- Toxic megacolon is a condition that occurs when the muscularis externa of the colon becomes involved by the inflammatory disease.
- The colon characteristically dilates to exceed six centimeters.
- This condition progresses rapidly and may become systemic.
- Toxic megacolon mandates aggressive treatment including:
  - Aggressive hydration
  - IV antibiotics
  - Gastric decompression
  - Elimination of anticholinergic drugs and other medications.
  - Surgical resection is recommended in selected cases.

Hemorrhoids

General
- Hemorrhoids are classified into two types according to their anatomical location.
- Hemorrhoids above the dentate line are internal hemorrhoids, whereas those below the dentate line are external hemorrhoids.

- Internal hemorrhoids are further classified into four different types.
  - 1st Degree hemorrhoids do not prolapse.
  - 2nd Degree hemorrhoids do prolapse but spontaneously reduce.
  - 3rd Degree hemorrhoids require manual reduction
  - 4th Degree hemorrhoids can not be reduced.

- The clinical presentation and treatment depends on the type of hemorrhoid.

- Risk factors associated with the development of symptomatic hemorrhoids are primarily the result of increased abdominal pressure such as constipation, excessive exercise, and pregnancy.

- Low-fiber diets may also play a role in the development of hemorrhoids.

- In addition, increased anal tone and portal hypertension are associated with hemorrhoid disease.

Clinical Manifestations
- **Internal hemorrhoids**
  - discomfort
  - bleeding
  - prolapse
- **External hemorrhoids**
  - pain (when they undergo thrombosis)
  - prolapse

Differential diagnosis
- Rectal prolapse
- Pruritus
- Cancer
- IBD
- STDs

Diagnosis
- History and physical examination
  - Inspection of the rectal and perineal area
- Examination with anoscope

Management

Medical treatment

- Internal hemorrhoids
    - 1st and 2nd degree hemorrhoids can be treated successfully medically
        1. Stool softeners
        2. Stool bulking agents
        3. Sitz baths
- External hemorrhoids
        1. Application of anesthetic ointment
        2. Sitz baths
        3. 1% hydrocortisone foam

Surgical treatment

- Internal hemorrhoids
    - 2nd-3rd degree hemorrhoids can be treated with rubber band ligation
    - Surgical resection is indicated for 4th if rubber band ligation is not possible
- External hemorrhoids
    - Surgical intervention is reserved for external hemorrhoids that present with bleeding or thrombosis.

The Appendix

Acute Appendicitis

General
- Appendicitis occurs due to inflammation of the appendix caused by occlusion of its lumen.
- Occlusion may be caused by hyperplasia of the lymphoid tissue (commonly seen in children) or by fecal material (fecalith), which is commonly seen in young adults.
- Acute appendicitis is the most common cause of acute abdomen.
- The age of onset is classically between 5-35 years old.
- In younger and older patients, the signs and symptoms of appendicitis are more insidious, which results in a higher rate of perforation. Thus, there is high degree of morbidity and mortality in these groups.

Clinical Manifestations
- **History**
  - Pain beginning in the periumbilical region and subsequently localizing to the **right lower quadrant** of the abdomen.
  - **Anorexia** (this is a reliable symptom of acute appendicitis)
  - Nausea and vomiting following the onset of pain.
- **Physical Exam**
  - Right lower quadrant tenderness (classically maximal point of tenderness occurs at **McBurney's point** which is one third of the distance from the anterior iliac spine to the umbilicus).
  - Low grade fever
  - Psoas sign (pain on extension of the right hip)
  - Obturator sign (pain on internal or external rotation of the hip)
  - Rovsing's sign (rebound palpation of the left lower quadrant produces pain in the right lower quadrant)
- The clinical findings of acute appendicitis may be different in patients with a retrocecal appendix, which occurs in over 15% of the cases.
- **Laboratory tests**
  - Leukocytosis (12,000-14,000 cells/μL)

Differential Diagnosis
- Stomach
  - Perforated ulcer
- Small bowel and appendix

- Meckel's diverticulum
- Intussusception
- SBO
• Cholecystitis
• Colon
  - Diverticulitis
  - Volvulus
  - Perforated viscus
  - Colon CA
  - IBD (Crohn's disease)
• Renal
  - UTI
  - Nephrolithiasis
• Ruptured AAA
• Gynecologic
  - Ectopic pregnancy
  - PID
  - Mittelschmerz
  - Ovarian torsion/cyst/tumor

Diagnosis

• **History and Physical Examination** is the most important element in determining the diagnosis of appendicitis. Thus, the diagnosis of acute appendicitis is a clinical one based signs and symptoms.

• **Leukocytosis** is also often used in the diagnosis of acute appendicitis. A general rule of thumb consists of making the diagnosis of acute appendicitis if two of the following three elements are present.

DIAGNOSIS OF APPENDICITIS (2 OF 3)

1. Right lower quadrant abdominal pain (must be present)

2. Good history (including anorexia)

3. Leukocytosis (12,000-14,000 cclls/μL)

• **Acute Abdominal Series.** If the diagnosis is still uncertain based on history and physical exam, an AAS may rule out a number of causes of abdominal pain present in the differential diagnosis.

• **In 5% of the cases a fecalith** can be observed in plain films. Plain films are also useful in assessing the possibility of perforation by noticing presence or absence of free air.

- **Urinalysis** is helpful in ruling out pyelonephritis. However, WBCs may be present in a patient with appendicitis.

- **Ultrasonography / CT-Scan** studies are helpful in determining degree of inflammation beyond the appendix and may assess presence of other pathology when the diagnosis of appendicitis is still not clear. This is especially the case in elderly patients where these tests are more helpful as they can also rule out other disease processes.

- **Barium Enema** is useful in children since it shows no filling of the appendix in appendicitis.

Treatment

- ABCs and appropriate resuscitation.

- Untreated appendicitis may lead to perforation in less than 24 h. Therefore, clinical suspicion of acute appendicitis requires prompt surgical intervention.

- Preoperative antibiotics to cover aerobic (and anaerobic is perforation is suspected) bacteria may be administered.

- Postoperative antibiotics for the first 24h if perforation has not occurred and for five to seven days in the case of perforation.

- If perforation is found intraoperatively, the incision is often allowed to close by secondary intention.

- An appendectomy should be performed even in the absence of an inflamed appendix. A 20% negative appendicitis rate is acceptable to prevent the risk of complication if appendicitis is missed.

- An appendectomy can also be performed laparoscopically. This procedure is even more desirable in the female patient when the diagnosis of appendicitis is not clear as gynecological pathology can be explored.

Cancer of the Appendix

General

- The most common type of cancer of the appendix is carcinoid tumor. These are cancers that originate from neuroectodermal cells.

- Thus, they are also known as APUDomas (amine precursor, uptake and decarboxylation).

- Since they have high potential for metastasis, APUDomas are considered malignant. These tumors produce large amounts of serotonin, which is responsible for the clinical manifestation when it reaches the systemic circulation.

- Serotonin is metabolized by the liver and the signs and symptoms may not be observed if serotonin encounters the liver before the systemic circulation.

Clinical Presentation
- Rarely presents as the carcinoid syndrome:
    - Cutaneous flushing
    - Bronchospasm and wheezing
    - Valvular heart disease → right sided heart failure
    - Chronic watery diarrhea

Diagnosis
- Most of the time it is an incidental finding during appendectomy
- Elevated serum serotonin
- Elevated 5-HIAA in the urine

Treatment
- **Surgical**
    - Appendectomy is usually performed if the tumor is less than 2 cm
    - Right hemicolectomy is performed if the carcinoid tumor is larger than 2 cm
- **Medical**
    - Octeotride infusion (somatostatin agonist)

Meckel's Diverticulum

General
- Meckel's diverticulum is a remnant of the embryonic vitelline duct, which connects the yolk sac to the primitive midgut in the embryo.
- It is the most common congenital anomaly of the small bowel.
- A number of characteristics can be remembered by the rule of 2's.
    - It is located 2 feet from the ileocecal valve
    - Symptoms develop in 2% of the patients
    - Incidence is 2% of the general population
    - There is a 2:1 male/female ratio
    - Symptoms usually occur before the age of 2

Clinical Presentation
- The clinical presentation is dependent on the number of complications that may occur secondary to a symptomatic Meckel's diverticulum.
- The following are common complications of symptomatic Meckel's diverticulum:

- Intestinal hemorrhage, especially in children. This usually occurs due to acid secretion from heterotopic gastric mucosa.

- Intestinal obstruction may present with abdominal pain, nausea, and vomiting

- Inflammation presents with abdominal pain similar to acute appendicitis

- Incarcerated/strangulated hernias (Littré's hernia)

Differential Diagnosis

- The differential diagnosis is that of right lower quadrant abdominal pain (see above)

Diagnosis

- The diagnosis is made primarily by history and physical examination.

- AAS may rule out other conditions of abdominal pain in the differential and lead more toward the diagnosis of Meckel's diverticulum.

- Barium and radionuclide studies may be required if there is suspicion of bleeding

Treatment

- Symptomatic Meckel's diverticulum should be resected.

    - Indications for resection of an asymptomatic diverticulum found incidentally are controvertial and include:
        - Presence of inflammation
        - Size > 2 inches long
        - Detection of heterotopic tissue
        - Attached mesodiverticular bands

Biliary Tract

General
The following are common lesions affecting the biliary tract:

LESIONS OF THE BILIARY TRACT

- **Cholelithiasis** is the formation of gallstones in the gallbladder.

- **Cholecystitis** is the obstruction of the cystic duct most commonly caused by gallstones that leads to infection of the gallbladder due to bile stasis. Acalculus cholecystitis occurs in about 10% of the cases of cholecystitis. It usually occurs in the hospitalized patient in whom stimuli to secrete bile has been impaired by prolonged fasting, TPN, trauma, or severe dehydration resulting in bile stasis and infection.

- **Empyema of the gallbaldder** is a complication of cholecystitis that results in the gallbladder filled with pus.

- **Choledocholithiasis** is complete or partial obstruction of the common bile duct (CBD) usually as a result of gallstones.

- **Cholangitis** is the obstruction of the CBD with infected non-draining bile behind the obstruction.

- **Suppurative Cholangitis** is the obstruction of the CBD with pus in the ducts under pressure.

- **Cholecystectomy** is the surgical removal of the gallbladder.
- **Cholecystostomy** is the surgical incision of the gallbladder with the evacuation of gallstones and external drainage placement. This procedure is indicated in patients who are poor surgical candidates.

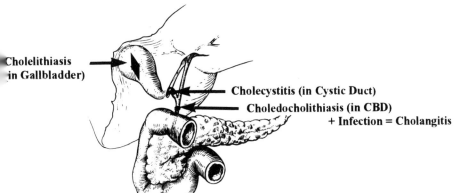

Cholelithiasis (in Gallbladder)

Cholecystitis (in Cystic Duct)

Choledocholithiasis (in CBD)
+ Infection = Cholangitis

Gallbladder and Common Bile Duct Disease

General
- The most common lesion affecting the gallbladder is cholelithiasis.
- Seventy-five percent of gallstones are made of cholesterol and 25% are made of bile pigments.
- Risk factors for the development of cholesterol stones are the classic four F's (Female, Fertile, Forty, Fat).
- The risk factors for bile pigments are hemolytic disorders, cirrhosis, and bile stasis.

Clinical Manifestations
- Eighty percent of biliary calculi are asymptomatic.

Symptomatic Calculi
- **Right upper quadrant pain**, usually described as **biliary colic**, which is **intermittent pain** in the right upper quadrant or epigastrium radiating to the back and scapula, often triggered by the ingestion of fatty foods.
- Nausea and vomiting
- Jaundice and sepsis may occur in complicated cases of cholelithiasis.

COMPLICATIONS OF CHOLELITHIASIS

- **Choledocholithiasis**
- **Cholangitis**
- **Gallstone pancreatitis**
- **Gallbladder necrosis**
- **Biliari-enteric fistulas** (biliary-duodenum, biliary-colon)
- **Gallstone ileus** occurs when a large gallstone migrates into the duodenum and causes small bowel obstruction, usually in the ileocecal valve.

Evaluation/Diagnosis
- History and physical examination
  - Biliary colic
  - Jaundice indicates obstruction of the biliary ducts.
  - **Murphy's sign** indicates inflammation of the gallbladder. This sign occurs when there is arrest of inspiration with palpation of the right upper quadrant.
  - **Charcot's Triad** suggests cholangitis and is associated with:

```
CHARCOT'S TRIAD
1. Fever/chills
2. Right upper quadrant pain
3. Jaundice
```

- **Reynolds's Pentad** is suggestive of acute suppurative cholangitis. It is Charcot's Triad plus altered mental status and shock.

• **Laboratory analysis**
  - Elevated WBC
  - Amylase/ lipase should be obtained to rule out gallstone pancreatitis
  - Bilirubin fractionation
  - LFTs (AST/ ALT, alkaline phosphatase). LFTs are useful in obtaining a good differential for elevated bilirubin.

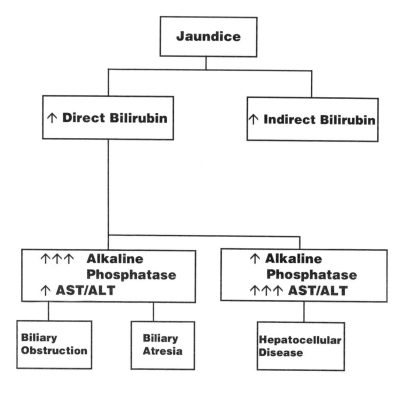

- Ultrasonography
  - Detects gallstones in 95% of the cases
  - Provides information on intra- and extrahepatic ducts
  - Suggests cholecystitis (gallstones, gallbladder wall thickening, fluid around gallbaldder)
  - It is not very sensitive to assess CBD dilatation (20% false negatives)
- Percutaneous transhepatic cholangiography (injection of contrast media directly into the intrahepatic duct) is most sensitive in delineating biliary anatomy and obstruction
- Radionucleide test (HIDA scan)—injection of technetium-99m IV concentrates in the bile and allows visualization of the biliary tree.
  - It is the definitive diagnosis for cholecystitis as it reveals obstruction in the cystic duct and can diagnose obstruction of the CBD.
- Endoscopic retrograde cholangiopancreatography (**ERCP**) is diagnostic and localizes for CBD obstruction

Treatment

- After assessment of ABCs and administration of analgesic medication, the treatment of biliary disease depends on the presentation and presence of complications.
- **Cholelithiasis**
  - Elective **cholecystectomy** is recommended for symptomatic cholelithiasis in the absence of complications and when the patient is a good surgical candidate.
  - **Cholecystectomy** for asymptomatic cholelithiasis in diabetic or immunocompromised patients is controversial. Sickle cell patients and children with large gallstones should also undergo elective **cholecystectomy**. Patients with calcified gallbladder (Porcelain gallbladder) have a 50% risk of developing carcinoma of the gallbladder and should have it removed.
  - **Cholecystectomy** can be performed by laparoscopic (**lap chole**) or open surgery. The laproscopic approach has less morbidity and mortality than open surgery, but is contraindicated in patients with prior right upper quadrant abdominal surgeries due to the possible presence of adhesions.
- **Cholecystitis**
  - NPO
  - Aggressive hydration
  - Antibiotics
  - Cholecystectomy (immediate vs. delayed)

- **Choledocholithiasis**
  - Cholecystectomy
  - **Intraoperative cholangiography (IOC)**—intraoperative injection of contrast material directly into the biliary ducts to clarify bile duct anatomy and localize stones.
  - Intraoperative common bile duct exploration (vertical incision is made in the CBD and the lumen is explored with a choledoscope) and T-tube placement.
  - The indications for a common bile duct exploration are:

INDICATIONS FOR COMMON BILE EXPLORATION	
Definitive indications	**Relative indications**
• Palpable CBD stone	• Duct dilatation
• CBD visualized by IOC	• Gallstone pancreatitis
• Cholangitis	• Recurrent jaundice
• Serum bilirubin > 7 mg/100 ml	• Small gallbladder stones
	• Biliary-enteric fistula

  - Retained CBD stones are managed by placement of a T-tube for longer duration (4-6 weeks) as CBD stones will spontaneously pass in 25% of the cases. If, by that time, the CBD stone has not passed, a repeat CBD exploration or ERCP with basket retrieval of the retained stone is recommended.
- **Cholangitis**
  - NPO
  - Aggressive hydration
  - Antibiotics
  - NG decompression
  - Cholecystectomy when patient is stable
- **Suppurative Cholangitis**
  - NPO
  - Aggressive hydration
  - Antibiotics
  - NG decompression
  - Emergent CBD decompression by ERCP, PTC or laparotomy
  - Cholecystectomy when patient is stable

The Pancreas

Acute Pancreatitis

General

- Acute pancreatitis occurs when there is a sudden inflammation of the pancreas caused by release and activation of pancreatic enzymes causing parenchymal destruction.
- The etiology of acute pancreatitis is not completely understood. However, several factors have been recognized as causes of acute pancreatitis.

Causes of Acute Pancreatitis

- Most of the causes of acute pancreatitis can be remembered by the mnemonic **BAD SHIT:**

B =	Biliary calculi
A =	Alcohol
D =	Drugs (furosemide, steroids, thiazides, estrogens)
S =	Scorpion bites (one of the least common causes of acute pancreatitis)
H =	Hyperparathyroidism ($\uparrow$ Ca^{++}) and hyperlipoproteinemias
I =	Infections (mumps, Coxsackie virus B, Epstein-Barr virus, rubella, hepatitis A and B)
T =	Trauma

- Biliary calculi and alcohol cause 85% of the cases of acute pancreatitis.
- The mechanism by which gallstones result in pancreatitis is not well understood.
- Obstruction of the ampulla of Vater and reflux of bile into the pancreatic duct are hypotheses that have been disproven by experimental data on animal models.
- Alcohol is thought to increase the protein secretory response of the pancreas. Perhaps precipitated proteins obstruct the pancreatic ducts.
- About 10% of the cases of acute pancreatitis are idiopathic.
- A complication of **ERCP** is acute pancreatitis in 1% of the cases and it is contraindicated in patients with a current episode of pancreatitis.

Complications of acute pancreatitis

- **Necrotizing pancreatitis** is a severe complication of acute pancreatitis occurring in about 15% of the cases. This may lead to bacterial superinfection and hemorrhagic pancreatitis (Cullen's sign occurs when there is bluish discoloration of the periumbilical area indicating hemorrhagic pancreatitis).

- **Pancreatic abscess** occurs in about 2% of the cases. It is the collection of purulent fluid around the pancreas. Antibiotics, percutaneous drain placement or operative debridement are the treatment options.

- Paralytic ileus

- **Pseudocysts** are cavities caused by the autodigestion of the pancreatic parenchyma. Pseudocyst formation is associated with inflammation, infection, obstruction and rupture. In acute pancreatitis, the amylase serum levels are initially elevated, but decrease with supportive management. Persistently elevated amylase should raise suspicion for pseudocyst formation.

Clinical Manifestations

- **History**
    - Constant epigastric pain radiating to the back
    - Nausea and vomiting
- **Physical examination**
    - Fever/ Tachycardia
    - Right upper and lower quadrant abdominal tenderness
    - Absent bowel sounds
    - Rebound tenderness
- **Laboratory**
    - Leukocytosis
    - Elevated amylase levels (sensitive test)
        - ✳ **Differential diagnosis of elevated amylase**
            - Liver disease
            - Salivary gland tumor/ inflammation/ trauma
            - SBO
            - Ruptured AAA
            - Pseudocyst
    - Elevated lipase levels (specific test)

Differential diagnosis of acute pancreatitis

- Stomach
    - PUD
    - Perforated ulcer
    - Gastritis
- Gallbladder
    - Cholelithiasis
    - Choledocholithiasis

- Cholecystitis
- Cholangitis
- Liver
  - Hepatic abscess
  - Liver tumors
  - Hepatitis
- Heart
  - Myocardial infarction
- Lungs
  - Pneumonia
  - PE
- Kidney
  - Pyelonephritis
  - Nephrolithiasis

Diagnosis

- History and physical examination (especially excessive alcohol use and biliary calculi)
- **Elevated amylase/lipase**
- Abdominal x-ray may reveal the following findings:
  - adynamic ileus
  - pancreatic calcifications
  - presence of gallstones (in 10% of cases)
- Ultrasonography (reveals inflammation and rules out complications)
  - gallstones (cholelithiasis)
  - pseudocyst
  - pancreatic abscess
- CT-scan (reveals inflammation and rules out complications)
  - pseudocyst
  - pancreatic abscess/ necrosis

Prognosis

- The prognosis of patients with acute pancreatitis can be assessed by the **Ranson criteria**.
- The Ranson/Imrie criteria can be remembered by the mnemonic **LAG WA** and **BOB CHS.**
- Of important note is that the **amylase level**, though diagnostic of pancreatitis, is not a prognostic factor of patient outcome with acute pancreatitis.
- The following table contains the factors associated with patient outcome with acute pancreatitis.

RANSON/IMRIE CRITERIA

At presentation	48 hours after presentation	Mortality
1) LDH > 350	1) Base excess > 4	• **0-2 < 5%**
2) AST > 250	2) pO_2 < 60 mm Hg	• **3-4 = 15%**
3) Glucose > 200	3) BUN increase > 5	• **5-6 = 40%**
4) WBC > 16,000	4) Ca^{++} < 8.0	• **7-8 = 100%**
5) Age > 55	5) Hct drop > 10%	
	6) Sequestered fluid > 6L	

Management

Medical
• ABCs
• NPO
• Aggressive fluid resuscitation
• Analgesia
• Hemodynamic and respiratory monitoring

Surgical
• Diagnostic uncertainty in the presence of hemodynamic instability is an indication for exploratory laparotomy.
• Pancreatitis secondary to biliary calculi—cholecystectomy alleviates pancreatitis and prevents recurrent attacks.
• Pancreatic drainage for necrotizing pancreatitis and pancreatic abscesses.

Chronic Pancreatitis

General
• Chronic pancreatitis occurs when there is permanent destruction of parenchyma of the pancreas resulting in fibrosis, calcification and loss of endocrine and exocrine pancreatic function.
• About 2% of patients with chronic pancreatitis develop **pancreatic cancer**.

Causes of Chronic Pancreatitis
• Alcohol
• Hyperparathyroidism (↑ Ca^{++})

- Hyperlipidemia
- Cystic fibrosis
- Familial pancreatitis
- Trauma
- Iatrogenic

Clinical Manifestations

- Epigastric intermittent pain associated with food ingestion
- Loss of exocrine function produces steatorrhea
- Loss of endocrine function produces signs and symptoms of diabetes

Diagnosis

- History and physical examination
- Amylase/lipase
- Stool fat analysis
- Glucose levels (serum/urine)
- CT scan
    - Demonstrates gland enlargement/atrophy, duct enlargement, calcification, masses, pseudocysts, inflammation or extension beyond the pancreas
- Ultrasonography is less sensitive than CT scan
- Abdominal x-ray demonstrates calcifications
- ERCP demonstrates ductal irregularities

Treatment

- **Medical Treatment**
    - Alcohol discontinuation
    - Treatment of the underlying disease (i.e., hypercalcemia)
    - Insulin for treatment of diabetes mellitus
    - Pancreatic enzyme replacement
- **Surgical Treatment**
    - Longitudinal pancreatojejunostomy (Puestow procdure)
    - Distal pancreatojejunostomy (Du Val procedure)
    - Near-total pancreatectomy

Pancreatic Carcinoma

General
- About 28,000 new cases/year in US
- 2:1 male: female ratio
- Greatest risk factors are age and cigarette smoking
- The most common type (90%) is poorly differentiated adenocarcinoma from the ductal epithelium
- 2/3 of cancers arise from the head of the pancreas
- Poor survival rate (5-10% 5-year survival rate after surgical intervention or biliary obstruction)

CLINICAL MANIFESTATIONS

Head of the pancreas	Body or tail
• Painless jaundice	• Nausea and vomiting
• Palpable nontender gall-bladder (Courvoisier's sign)	• Weight loss and fatigue
• Pruritus	• Migratory thrombophlebitis
• Dark urine	• Jaundice
• ↑ Direct bilirubin	
• ↑ Alkaline phosphatase	

Diagnosis
- History and physical examination
- Elevated bilirubin/alkaline phosphatase (indicates biliary obstruction)
- Abdominal CT-scan
- Ultrasonography
- ERCP with biopsy

Treatment
- Body and tail of the pancreas
    - Distal resection of the pancreas
- Head of the pancreas
    - **Whipple** procedure (5% mortality rate)
        1. **Cholecystectomy**
        2. **Arterectomy with truncal vagotomy**
        3. **Pancreaticoduodenectomy** (resection of the head of the pancreas and duodenum).

4. **Choledochojejunostomy** (anastamosis of the common bile duct to the jejunum).
5. **Pancreaticojejunostomy** (anastamosis of the distal pancreas to the jejunum).
6. **Gastrojejunostomy** (anastamosis of the stomach to the jejunum).

WHIPPLE PROCUDURE

Three resections

1. Head of the pancreas ⟶
2. Stomach ⟶
3. Gall bladder ⟶

} Jejunum

Three anastamoses

1. Pancreaticojejunostomy
2. Gastrojejunostomy
3. Choledochojejunostomy

4 | VASCULAR SURGERY

Vascular System Disease

Atherosclerosis
General
- Atherosclerosis is the focal narrowing of vessels that result in intimal proliferation of the smooth muscle cells of the arterial wall and the deposition of lipids. In later stages calcifications also occur.
- Atherosclerosis is responsible for most of the vascular pathology encountered by the surgeon.
- Understanding sequelae of this disease is important as patients with vascular disease have many co-morbid conditions which could complicate surgical interventions.

Risk Factors for Atherosclerosis
- Age
- Hypertesion
- Diabetes mellitus
- Hyperlipedemia
- Smoking
- Family history of atherosclerosis

Consequences of Atherosclerosis
The typical sequelae of atherosclerosis is indicated by the arrow below. The left side of the arrow indicates early stages of the disease and right indicates complications that are seen as the disease progresses:

Heart	Extracranial Vascular Disease	Peripheral Vascular Disease Disease
• Coronry artery disease	• Transient ischemic attack	• Intermittent claudication
• Angina	• Reversible ischemic	• Rest pain
• Myocardial infarction	neurologic defect	• Gangrene
	• Cerebrovascular accident	

Coronary Artery Disease (CAD)

- CAD is the progressive narrowing or occlusion of the coronary arteries due to atherosclerosis.
- The risk factors for the development of CAD are identical to the ones for atherosclerosis.
- The complications of CAD are **angina** and **myocardial infarction**.

Angina Pectoris

General
- Angina is substernal chest pain or pressure that occurs when there is increased demand for oxygen and nutrients by the myocardium as in exercise or anxiety.
- When the symptoms occur at rest or when there are changes in symptoms, more severe narrowing has occurred and this is referred to as **unstable angina**.
- **Variant angina or Prinzmetal's angina** is the occurrence of symptoms due to vasospasm of the coronary arteries. Thus, the symptoms may also occur at rest or while sleeping. The etiology of the vasospasm is not well understood.

Clinical Manifestations
- Chest pain or pressure due to atherosclerotic narrowing of the coronary arteries.
- There is no correlation between the degree of narrowing and the severity of chest pain.

Diagnosis
- **History and physical examination**
- **ECG** changes which are usually S-T segment depression and Q wave inversion during the symptomatic period.
- Relief of symptoms by use of **nitroglycerin** within minutes is almost always diagnostic of angina.
- **Exercise stress test**.
  - This test is performed on a stationary bicycle or treadmill. A slope can be adjusted to increase workload. Symptoms (chest pain, dizziness, shortness of breath) and signs (heart rate, blood pressure, and EKG) are recorded with increasing amounts of workload. This test is usually able to reproduce the symptoms of angina.
- **Stress test with thallium scan** is indicated when the diagnosis is not obvious with the above tests or with the asymptomatic patient (i.e. diabetic patient) with a high degree of suspicion.
  - Thallium accumulates in normal cells. This radioactive substance can be detected in normal cells. Areas of ischemic or necrotic tissue will be unlabeled on the scan.

- **Gated radionuclide scans.**
  - In this tests red blood cells are labeled and pictures of the heart are taken to detect motion abnormalities.
- Caridiac catheterization is the gold standard for the diagnosis of CAD.
  - In this test, a catheter is advanced to the coronary ostium and a dye is injected into the lumen of the coronary vessels. The picture taken, therefore, reveals the luminal architecture of the coronary vessels. Even though this test is the gold standard for CAD, it is not performed routinely due to the potential risk of complications, which include stroke, myocardial infarction and death.

Management

Medical Management
- Reduction of risk factors for CAD is an important modality in the management of angina.
- Pharmacological treatment includes:
  - Nitrates
  - Pain management
  - β-blockers
  - Ca^{++} channel blockers (preferred treatment for variant angina)

- Percutaneous transluminal coronary angioplasty (**PTCA**) is a technique in which a balloon in inserted to the affected vessel and inflated to relieve the stenosis. This is indicated for patients with single vessel involvement. This modality is associated with high restenosis and carries complications of MI, complete obstruction of the vessel, and rupture.

Surgical Management:
- Coronary Artery Bypass Graft Surgery (**CABG**) is indicated for patients with disease of the left main coronary artery or for patients with three-vessel disease.
- Two graft vessels are usually used for replacement or bypass of the diseased coronary vessels:
  - **Shaphenous vein** grafts have up to 60% patency after 10 years
  - **Internal mammary artery (IMA)** grafts have over 90% patency after 10 years.
  - Radial arteries are sometimes used.

Myocardial Infarction (MI)

General
- MI usually occurs due to an acute obstruction of a coronary artery by an embolus or a thrombus. This is almost always due to atherosclerosis.

Clinical Manifestations
- Symptoms of angina of longer duration

- Anxiety
- Diaphoresis
- Tachycardia
- Shortness of breath
- Nausea and vomiting
- Syncope

Clinical manifestations suggestive of complications

- **Anterior MI** (LAD coronary artery) may present with symptoms of left ventricular failure:
    - Ventricular arrhythmias
    - Cardiogenic shock:
        - Pulmonary edema
        - Hypotension
        - Oliguria
        - Confusion
- **Inferior MI** (RCA) may present with complete heart block and parasympathetic manifestations such as bradycardia.

Diagnosis

- History and physical examination
- ECG changes:
    - T wave inversion
    - S-T segment elevation
    - Q waves
- Indicative laboratory tests
    - CK-MB
    - LDH
    - SGOT
    - Troponin I
- Echocardiogram
- Thallium scans → can localize the infarction
- Cardiac catheterization
- If two of the following tests are positive, one should have a high degree of suspicion for A or I
    - chest pain
    - EKG changes
    - increased troponin I

Management

- ABCs
- Pain management
- Antiarrhythmic prophylaxis (lidocaine, procainamide)
- Thrombolytic agents
    - Urokinase
    - Tissue plasminogen activator (t-PA)
- PTCA
- CABG

Cerebrovascular Insufficiency

General

- Cerebrovascular disease may be caused by several pathologic processes involving the vasculature of the brain.

- The process may be intrinsic to the vessel (atherosclerosis), may originate remotely (an embolus from the heart), may be due to inadequate cerebral blood flow (an acute hypotensive episode), or may result from a ruptured blood vessel.

- The differential diagnosis for cerebrovascular insufficiency is complex. The most common causes of cerebrovascular insufficiency encountered by the vascular surgeon include:

  - Atherosclerotic narrowing of the carotid or vertebral circulation
    - Atherosclerosis of the cerebrovascular system may lead to cerebrovascular insufficiency in two ways:
      - **Thromboembolism from carotid bifurcation** is by far the most common cause of symptoms.
      - Progressive narrowing of carotid or vertebral vessels resulting in hypoperfusion occurs much less commonly than the above.

    - The clinical manifestations of atherosclerosis of the carotid arteries have similar anatomical distribution in repeated episodes.

  - **Emboli of cardiac origin** occur most frequently due to atrial fibrillation, with varying symptoms relating to anatomic location of embolus.

Clinical Manifestations

- The clinical manifestations of cerebrovascular insufficiency are neurological deficits, which depend on the area of the brain affected and on the compensatory capacity of the dual circulation at the circle of Willis.

- Ischemic stroke is a clinical manifestation that results due to cerebrovascular insufficiency.

- Approximately 80 percent of strokes are due to ischemic cerebral infarction while 20 percent are due to brain hemorrhage.

- The clinical manifestations of ischemic stroke depend on the arterial tree affected.

- Two main arteries supply the brain:

- **Internal Carotid Artery (ICA)**
- **Vertebral Arteries (VA)**

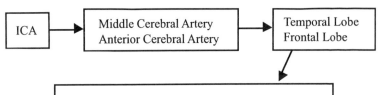

Most often the middle cerebral artery is involved resulting in contralateral weakness and sensory loss, which is pronounced **in the face. Speech area** may be affected if the left side is involved. If the anterior cerebral artery is involved, **sensory motor deficits** of the leg and foot result. Occasionally the ophthalamic artery is affected leading to temporary blindness on the ipsilateral side. **(amaurosis fugax)**

- Transient blindness occurs commonly due to thromboembolism from the carotid arteries. It may also occur by occlusion of the ophthalmic artery. This event is referred to as **amaurosis fugax**, an opthalmic TIA (see below).

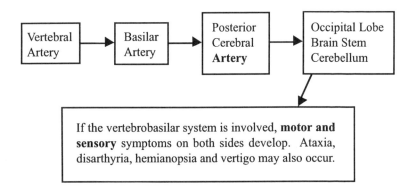

If the vertebrobasilar system is involved, **motor and sensory** symptoms on both sides develop. Ataxia, disarthyria, hemianopsia and vertigo may also occur.

The duration of the neurological defect may be variable:
- Transit ischemic attack **(TIA)** is a neurological deficit that completely resolves in 24 hours. However, TIAs usually last for only a few minutes. Opthalamic artery TIAs result in **amaurosis fugax**.

- Reversible ischemic neurological deficit **(RIND)** is a neurological defect that takes 1-7 days for complete resolution. This term is currently falling into disfavor.

- Cerebrovascular accident (**CVA**) is a neurological defect that takes more than one week to resolve or causes permanent neurological damage.

Diagnosis

- **History and physical examination**
  - History of angina, risk factors for atherosclerosis
  - Physical examination should check for presence of carotid bruits. Not all advanced plaques produce bruits.
- **Carotid ultrasound/doppler** provides information on the degree of stenosis.
- **CT-Scan without IV** contrast detects infarction and hemorrhage.
- **MRI** is the most sensitive test for evaluation of infarction or hemorrhage.
- **Arteriogram** is the gold standard of cerebrovascular disease and is done selectively on patients considered for surgery.

Management

- ABCs
- A patient diagnosed with a TIA, RIND, or CVA should be admitted to the hospital to establish the source of the thrombus/embolus and for appropriate management.

- **Medical management**
  - Thrombolytic agents (urokinase, t-PA) may be used for the treatment of acute stroke.
  - Anticoagulation therapy (heparin/warfarin) is controversial and depends on the size and source of the embolus/thrombus, as well as other risk factors.
  - Prophylactic treatment with antiplatelet agents and coumadin may also be employed in certain patients who have no risk factors for bleeding.
  - Reduction of risk factors is an important element in the management of cerebrovascular disease.
- **Surgical treatment**
  - Carotid endarterectomy (**CEA**) is the removal of the tunica intima and media of the affected carotid artery. This operation carries a 1% mortality risk due to CVA, MI, or intracranial hemorrhage.
  - CEA is recommended in the asymptomatic patient with > 70% stenosis as the risk for the development of a CVA is about 5%.
  - CEA is indicated for the asymptomatic patient with > 70% stenosis or 50% stenosis in the symptomatic patient with multiple TIAs.
  - CEA is contraindicated in patients with severe permanent neurological damage.

Peripheral Vascular Disease (PVD)

General
- Peripheral vascular disease (PVD) refers to the narrowing of the arteries of the lower extremities due to atherosclerosis, but can also affect upper extremities or viscera.

Clinical Manifestations
- **Intermittent Claudication** is a clinical syndrome associated with pain of large muscle groups that occurs during exercise and is relieved by rest.
    - This occurs as a result of inadequate blood flow to the muscle during increased metabolic demand.
    - The clinical manifestations occur below the level of occlusion:
    - Aortoiliac occlusive disease is associated with claudication of the buttocks.
        - This may be associated with buttock atrophy and impotence (Leriche's syndrome). These patients also usually present with calf cramps as well.
    - Superficial femoral artery occlusion causes **calf claudication**. This is the most common site affected in PVD.
    - Intermittent claudication has the following characteristics:

> 1. **Pain** with increased activity of the affected muscle group.
>
> 2. **Reproducibility**: muscle pain occurs in roughly the same location with the same amount of exercise each time.
>
> 3. **Pain is relieved by rest**.

    - Intermittent claudication carries a 5% risk of major amputation or gangrene in 5 years without treatment. The poor outcome of these patients is also due to other diseases, e.g., diabetes mellitus.
- **Rest pain** is a more serious condition in the sequelae of PVD.
    - Rest pain refers to the pain of the toes and forefoot at rest.
    - This usually occurs at night. At night patients do not have the hydrostatic component of the upright position. Also during sleep the cardiac

output is decreased. These conditions further compromise oxygen and nutrient delivery to the affected muscle group.

- Standing or hanging the foot on the side of the bed relieves the pain.

- About 50% of the patients with rest pain will have complications of gangrene in five years and will require amputation if left untreated.

Signs of PVD:

- Decreased peripheral pulses
- ↓ sweating
- Atrophy of the skin
- Hair loss
- Bruits
- Thick toe nails
- Blanching of the skin
- **Ulcers**:
  - The severe ischemia to the lower extremity causes changes in the skin and may result in an arterial ulcer.
  - **Arterial ulcers** are characterized by pain with a distribution over the lower third of the dorsum of the foot or on the toes. The presence of an arterial ulcer is a high risk factor for **gangrene**. **Wet gangrene** is of particular concern as it as it indicates infection that can rapidly ascend. **Dry gangrene** represents tissue necrosis without active infection.
  - **Venous ulcers** are located around the ankle and are not as painful.
  - **Diabetic ulcers** are similar to arterial ulcers in distribution but are characteristically painless. These often occur at pressure points such as the metatarsal head, or friction points caused by shoes.

Diagnosis

- History and physical examination
- Doppler recordings
  - A hand-held Doppler device may assess the degree of occlusion. Normal recordings display a triphasic wave form. With progression of the disease, this wave changes from triphasic to biphasic to monophasic, which indicates severe occlusion.
  - Ankle to brachial index (**ABI**) is the ratio of the systolic blood pressure at the ankle to that of the brachial artery. The pressure is determined by Doppler to increase sensitivity of the recording.

- **ABI   1.0 → Normal**
- **ABI < 0.95 → Claudication**
- **ABI < 0.4 → Rest pain**

- Patients with longstanding diabetes mellitus may have falsely elevated ABIs due to calcified arterial walls.

- **Arteriogram** is the gold standard to establish the diagnosis of PVD. Arteriogram is not required to establish the diagnosis as this can be obtained reliably from the H&P. However, an arteriogram maps the disease, which is important to determine treatment options.

Management
The management of PVD depends on the severity of the disease.

- The treatment of **intermittent claudication** is conservative.

  - An **important modality** for the management of claudication is the reduction of risk factors for PVD.

    1. Cessation of tobacco use
    2. Weight loss in obese patients
    3. Exercise

  - Arteriodilators **do not** improve symptoms as patients with PVD have exhausted the arterial compensatory mechanisms to maximize blood flow.
  - **Pentoxifylline** ameliorates the symptoms of claudication by increasing RBC deformability, facilitating passage through arterial stenosis. This works in about one third of the patients and should be employed only after aggressive conservative management has failed.
  - **Bypass surgery** is reserved for patients with severe claudication who have failed all conservative modalities. Limb-threat patients should also undergo bypass surgery.

- **Rest pain** mandates more aggressive intervention.
  - Transluminal balloon angioplasty uses a catheter to dilate the diseased artery. Patient selection for transluminal balloon angioplasty should be

similar to those patients being considered for surgery.

- Endarterectomy is the treatment of choice for carotid artery occlusion, but has a more limited role in the management of PVD. The affected area of the carotid is usually short. In contrast, in PVD, longer segments are affected or the disease is caused by occlusion.

- Patients who develop symptoms of rest pain should be considered for bypass surgery, the treatment of choice for PVD. Other indications for bypass surgery include:

    1. Limb-threat
    2. Wet gangrene
    3. Tissue necrosis

Common bypass interventions:

• Femoral-popliteal (FEM-POP) bypass uses an autologous (saphenous) or prosthetic vein graft to bypass the superficial femoral artery occlusion from the femoral artery to the popliteal artery.

• Femoral distal bypass uses an autologous (saphenous) or prosthetic vein grafted from the femoral artery to a distal artery such as the peroneal or anterior/posterior tibial arteries.

• Aortobifemoral bypass uses the infrarenal aorta anastamosed to common femoral arteries or superficial femoral artery if patent.

• Extra-anatomic subcutaneous bypass surgery (axillofemoral, femorofemoral) is preferred in patients who are at high risk of abdominal surgical interventions. Complications from this procedure are more frequent due to the longer course of the graft and possibility of subcutaneus compressions.

Deep Venous Thrombosis (DVT) and Pulmonary Thromboembolism (PTE)

General

- DVT and PTE are related disorders that are commonly encountered by the vascular surgeon and are potentially life-threatening.
- Any DVT can propagate and embolize. A common site of embolization is the lungs, which results in obstruction of pulmonary vasculature and is responsible for the clinical manifestations of pulmonary thromboembolism.
- The vast majority of potentially life-threatening DVTs originate from the deep venous system of the thighs.
- The clinical manifestations of DVT and PTE are nonspecific. Therefore, the surgeon must be aware of potential risk factors for the development of any of these conditions.
- Common risk factors are described by the **Virchow's triad**:

> 1. Trauma to the blood vessel.
> 2. Venous stasis
> 3. Increased blood coagulability

- Patients who present with any factors present in the Virchow's triad are at an increased risk for the development of DVT and PTE.
- **Risk factors for venous stasis**
    - Prolonged bed rest
        - After surgery
        - Long travel
    - Pregnancy increases venous stasis in the pelvic veins
    - Varicose veins result in valvular incompetence and stasis
    - Cardiac disease
- **Increased blood coagulability**
    - Pregnancy increases clotting factors
        - Estrogens
        - Birth control pills
    - Obesity
    - Hematological disorders
    - Cancer

Clinical Manifestations

Clinical manifestations of DVT

- Leg pain
- Leg swelling

- Erythema
- Tenderness
- **Homans' sign** is tenderness of the calf muscles with dorsiflexion of the foot.

Clinical manifestations of PTE
- **Acute onset of dyspnea**
- **Tachypnea**
- Tachycardia
- Rales
- Pleuritic chest pain
- Hypotension and right-sided ventricular heave indicates massive PTE and requires aggressive treatment
- EKG changes include:
  - Sinus tachycardia
  - Atrial fibrillation
  - S-T wave changes
- **Arterial blood gases**
  - Hyperventilation
  - ↑ Aa gradient
    - Aa gradient = $(150 - pCO_2/0.8)$-pO_2
    - Normal Aa gradient = $age/4 + 4$

Diagnosis

Diagnosis of DVT
- High degree of suspicion based on history, physical examination and associated risk factors.
- **Doppler ultrasound** detects changes of interrupted blood flow. Differences in blood flow in both legs is noted. Bilateral DVTs are uncommon.
- **Duplex sonography** is a technique that combines doppler flow through the venous system of the venous system and direct ultrasound of the clot. This is an excellent diagnostic tool for DVT as it may reveal:
  1. ↓ blood flow
  2. clot formation
  3. **interrupted blood flow**
- **Impedance plethysmography** is a technique that measures maximal venous output and venous capacitance. A patient with DVT has lower capacitance due to edema in the leg.
- **Contrast venography** is the gold standard for the diagnosis of DVTs and reveals filling defects due to narrowing of the vessels by the clot. This technique is more invasive and carries more morbidity.

Diagnosis of PTE
- History and physical examination
- EKG changes
- Arterial blood gases
- Ventilation-perfusion (V/Q) scan
- Pulmonary angiogram

Treatment
- Diagnosis or high suspicion of DVT mandates immediate anticoagulation in patients who have no contraindications.
- This is usually started with heparin and followed with warfarin.
- The treatment for PTE is the same as for DVT.
- Hypotensive patients or patients in shock should be considered for immediate **embolectomy** as these signs suggest massive PTE and the mortality rate is high.

Aneurysms

- Aneurysms may also be a complication of atherosclerosis.
- Even though the etiology of aneurysm is thought to be multifactorial, atherosclerosis is present in over 90% of the cases.
- There are certain congenital vascular disorders that have a predisposition for the formation of aneurysms, e.g., Marfan's syndrome.
- An aneurysm is defined as **dilation of an artery 1.5-2 times its normal diameter**. There are two main types of aneurysms:
    - **True aneurysms** are aneurysms composed of all layers of the arterial wall.
    - **False aneurysms** are usually the result of trauma. They do not involve all layers of the arterial wall and are composed of a fibrous capsule.
- Mycotic aneurysm is a rare type of aneurysm that occurs as a result of damaged produced by a fungal infection of the arterial wall.
- The following are common sites for the formation of aneurysms:

    1. Infrarenal abdominal aorta
    2. Common femoral arteries
    3. Popliteal artery

Abdominal Aortic Aneurysm (AAA)

General
- AAA occurs when dilation of abdominal aorta is > 1.5 times its normal diameter.

- The most common site affected is the infrarenal aorta.

Clinical Presentation

- The clinical presentation of **AAA** is usually asymptomatic until complications from the aneurysm develop.

- Signs in the asymptoamtic patient include a **pulsatile abdominal mass**, and **abdominal bruits**.

- Complications of **AAA** include:

  1. Rupture
  2. Severe abdominal or back pain due to extesion of the aneurysm
  3. Embolization (uncommon)
  4. Thrombosis (very rare)

Rupture of an **AAA** is a surgical emergency and requires immediate surgical intervention. A ruptured **AAA** classically presents with a the following triad:

> - **Very severe abdominal pain radiating to the back**
> - **Pulsatile abdominal mass**
> - **Hypotension**

- Aortic dissection is usually not a complication of an aneurysm. This is a separate condition in which the tunica media of the vessel (usually thoracic aorta) is ruptured, and creates a second lumen. This condition may also be a surgical emergency.

Diagnosis

- History and physical examination
  - Risk factors for PVD
  - Bruits, pulsatile mass
  - Hypotension
- Ultrasound
- CT-scan
- Plain abdominal x-rays may detect calcified aneurysms.
- Aortogram is not useful to establish the presence of an aneurysm as the luminal diameter is independent of the size of an aneurysm.

Management

- There is no medical management for the treatment of aneurysms. Reduction of risk factors may slow but not prevent growth of an aneurysm.

- A symptomatic AAA is a life-threatening condition and requires immediate surgical intervention. The diseased aorta is dissected and replaced with a prosthetic graft. The prosthetic material is usually covered on its entire surface with the sac of the native aneurysm to prevent fistula formation. The mortality of a ruptured AAA when the diagnosis is delayed is nearly 100%.
- Surgical treatment for an asymptomatic AAA depends on the size of the aneurysm, the rate of growth and medical condition of the patient.

> - **AAAs grow at rate of 2-4 mm per year**
> - **A patient with a AAA > 5cm should be considered for surgery**
> - **The risk of rupture for a AAA > 5cm is 30% in 3 years**
> - **Symptomatic AAAs (those presenting with abdominal pain, back pain, and hypotension) have a risk of rupture of 30% in 1 month.**

Complications
- Elective repair of an unruptured AAA carries a 2% mortality rate
- Ruptured AAAs carry a 50% operative mortality rate.
- Myocardial infarction
- Renal failure
- Colonic ischemia
- Aortoenteric fistula is a late complication

Aortic Dissection

General
- Aortic dissection occurs when the intima of the aorta is damaged creating a second lumen for blood flow.
- Aortic dissection is usually secondary to long-standing hypertension.
- Congenital vascular disorders may also predispose the patient to the formation of an aortic dissection.
- There are three types of dissections that are distinguished by their location along the aorta.
  - **Type I** occurs in the ascending aorta and involves the great vessels. This usually occurs in the patient with long standing hypertension.

- **Type II** has the same location but does not involve the great vessels. Type II dissection is common in the patient with congenital vascular disease.

- **Type III** occurs in the descending aorta and usually occurs due to atherosclerosis.

Clinical Manifestations

• Sharp stabbing pain radiating to the back is a common clinical presentation.

• The clinical manifestations of an aortic dissection depend on the type.

   - Type I may present as MI or CVA with the associated symptoms of each.

   - Type II and III dissections usually carry fewer complications.

• Visceral (renal or mesenteric) insufficiency or extremity insufficiency resulting from occlussion of the aortic branches by dissection.

Diagnosis

• History and physical examination

• Chest x-ray may demonstrate a widened mediastinum

• Aortography is the gold standard

Management

• Type I and II require immediate surgery with dissection of the diseased aorta with replacement by a prosthetic graft

• Type III may respond well to medical management and consists of control of hypertension, unless there is severe visceral or extremity insufficienfy.

5 | BREAST DISEASE

Breast Disease

General

- The female breast is composed of glandular, ductal, connective, and fatty tissue.
- **Fibroglandular** tissue refers to the composite of dense fibrous stroma and functional lobules and ducts.
- The 12-14 lobules in each breast are responsible for milk production, which is carried to the nipple by the array of ducts. These structures are supported by the stroma composed of connective tissue (**Cooper's ligaments**) and fat.
- During the reproductive years, the amount of fibroglandular tissue predominates over fat. Fibroglandular tissue **responds to estrogen and progesterone**. This is responsible for breast changes seen during the menstrual cycle.
- After menopause, the fibroglandular tissue begins to **involute** and is **replaced by fat**, which makes mammography more sensitive.
- The major lymphatic drainage of the breast is to the axilla.
- A minor drainage occurs to the parasternal nodes, which run with the internal mammary artery.
- Supraclavicular and contralateral nodes are not within the normal path of lymphatic drainage.
- In women who present to the physician with a breast mass, the following distribution of breast conditions is observed.

PERCENTAGE OF BREAST CONDITIONS IN WOMEN WITH A BREAST MASS

Conditions of the Breast	Percentage
Fibrocystic Changes	40%
No disease	30%
Benign tumors	13%
Cancer	10%
Fibroadenoma	7%

Benign Breast Masses

Fibrocystic Changes

- Fibrocystic changes refers to (usually several) painful masses in the breast.
- The pain and masses are often bilateral.
- The masses may be caused by any of the following:

FIBROCYSTIC CHANGES

1. Cyst formation
2. Glandular or connective tissue hyperplasia
3. Lymphatic infiltration
4. Stromal fibrosis
5. Apocrine metaplasia or hyperplasia
6. Sclerosing adenosis

- Fibrocystic changes are the **most common** lesions affecting the female breast, most often in the 30-50- year-old group.
- One of **the hallmarks of fibrocystic changes is its cyclic nature,** which is usually associated with monthly breast tenderness. This may be due to the physiological response of fibroglandular tissue to menstrual hormonal changes as breast engorgement and tenderness occur immediately before or during menstruation.
- Most fibrocystic changes do not have an associated risk for cancer.
- The management of fibrocystic changes is conservative and consists of:

TREATMENT OF FIBROCYSTIC CHANGES

1. Regular follow up and symptomatic treatment for tenderness.
2. Decreasing caffeine intake
3. Reduction of tobacco use
4. Vitamin E has been advocated to decrease the incidence of fibrocystic changes.
5. If a distinct mass associated with fibrocystic changes is present, ultrasound can usually be used to differentiate between cystic or solid masses.
6. If uncertainty still exists, cyst aspiration is indicated. Cysts usually disappear following aspiration.
7. Solid masses or a bloody aspirate require further work up.

Fibroadenomas

General

- Fibroadenomas are encapsulated fibromas that are easily recognized on physical examination by their specific character consisting of a well defined, smooth, firm, movable mass.
- They usually occur in the 20-30 year-old age group.
- Fibroadenomas also respond to hormonal stimulation and may grow during pregnancy.
- There is no risk of malignancy with fibroadenomas and these may be followed conservatively. Surgical excision is an alternative option as fibroadenomas can grow and some may develop into cystosarcoma phyllodes.

Breast Cancer

General

- One in eight women will develop breast cancer in their lifetime.
- Risk factors for carcinoma of the breast include:

RISK FACTORS FOR BREAST CANCER

1. Age
2. **Radiation exposure**
3. **History of breast or breast-ovarian cancer in first-degree relatives** (mother, sister, daughter). However, only about 10% of all breast cancers appear to be familial.
4. Two genes associated with familial breast cancer have been identified, **BRCA-1 and BRCA-2**. Patients with these genes have an 85% lifetime risk of developing breast cancer.
5. Early menarche
6. **Nulliparity or late child bearing** also appear to be minor risk factors in the development of breast cancer.

Clinical Presentation/ Symptoms and signs

Symptoms	Signs
• Asymptomatic • Breast mass (most common presentation) • Nipple retraction and discharge • Edema	• Mass (palpable range > 1 cm) • Edema • Lymphadenopathy: axillary (the most common metastasis) supraclavicular (indicates poor prognosis)

Evaluation

• History and physical examination.

• The table below indicates some important information that should be obtained with the H&P.

History	Physical
1. **Age** (80% of breast cancer occurs after age 40) 2. **Family history** of breast or ovarian cancer. 3. **Gynecological history** including age of onset of menses and/or menopause, gravidy, parity, age at first pregnancy, hormone therapy, and oral contraceptive use. 4. **Previous history** of abnormal mammograms, breast cancer, or fibrocystic changes. If a **mass** is **present**, information on the duration, character, possible monthly changes and pain should be obtained.	1. **Observe**: breast symmetry, skin changes (edema, discoloration, ulceration, or thickening), nipple discharge or retraction. 2. **Palpate**: establish location and character of the mass (firm, regular, movable, size), determine if there is tenderness with palpation, assess lymphadenopathy (axillary, supraclavicular).

- Any breast mass requires a prompt diagnosis.
- If a mass is suspected to be cystic by H&P, aspiration should be performed.
- If it does not disappear, it should be biopsied.
- **Diagnosis is made by tissue biopsy.**
- Benign breast disease does not require a specific diagnosis, but biopsy may be indicated to exclude malignancy.
- There are several tools available to the surgeon in the evaluation of a breast mass, though tissue biopsy is the only **definitive diagnostic tool**.

Mammography

- Mammograms are radiologic images of the breast, which are used for screening purposes in the asymptomatic patient over the age of 40.
- In the symptomatic patient, they only increase or decrease the suspicion of cancer and may be used to evaluate the contralateral breast and different areas of the ipsilateral breast.
- Mammography can also be used to guide the surgeon to obtain a biopsy in non-palpable masses.
- Other forms of screening include breast self-examination (BSE) and physical examination by a physician.
- The American Cancer Society recommendations for breast cancer screening are as follows:

Age	Screening /frequency
>20	Monthly self-examination
20-40	Physical examination every 3 years
>40	Physical examination every year
40-50	Mammogram every other year
>50	Mammogram every year

Ultrasonography

- Ultrasound is a noninvasive test that can quickly discriminate between solid and cystic masses.

Fine-needle aspiration (FNA)

- FNA is a sensitive technique for diagnosing breast cancer.
- Aspirated cells are smeared on a slide and cytologic evaluation is performed.
- It is possible to assess the grade (the degree to which tumor cells resemble normal cells).

• One of the limitations of FNA is that it can not assess tumor invasion. Thus, further tests are required.

Core-needle biopsy:

• Core-needle biopsy removes several cores of tissue with a 14-gauge needle preserving tissue architecture, which provides information about tumor invasion. If enough tissue is not available for diagnosis, excisional biopsy is required.

Excisional biopsy

• Excisional biopsy involves the complete removal of the mass and is usually performed under local anesthesia.

Stereotactic biopsy

• Stereotactic biopsy is a procedure in which small samples of tissue are removed from the breast using a hollow needle.

• The needle is carefully guided to the suspicious location by mammography and the use of computer coordinates.

Common Types of Breast Cancer

• About 90% of breast cancers arise from the ductal system.

• The remaining 10% arise from the lobules. Thus, breast cancers are either named ductal or lobular.

• The following table describes different types of breast cancers and their frequency.

Breast Cancer	% Frequency of occurrence
Infiltrating ductal CA	
Pure	53
Combined with other types	22
Medullary Carcinoma	6.0
Combined lobular and ductal CA	6.0
Infiltrating lobular CA	5.0
Colloid CA	2.3
Paget's disease	2.0

Lobular carcinoma *in situ* (LCIS)

- LCIS is a noninvasive type of cancer. Women with LCIS have a nine fold higher risk of developing breast cancer than the general population, with the cancer occurring in either breast.
- These lesions are usually picked up as incidental findings as there are rarely signs and symptoms.
- Treatment consists of close follow up.

Ductal carcinoma *in situ* (DCIS)

- DCIS is also known as intraductal carcinoma.
- These tumors usually do no cause distant metastasis, but can infiltrate the ductal system and produce extensive lesions.
- Comedo carcinoma is a subtype of intraductal carcinoma, which is characterized by high-grade histology.
- These cancers are thought to be precursors for invasive cancer, with the cancer occurring in the same breast.
- Treatment consists of excision with or without radiation.

Infiltrating (invasive) ductal carcinoma

- Invasive ductal carcinoma is the most common type of malignancy of the female breast.
- Because of its hard consistency due to the increased fibrous tissue stroma, this type of cancer is also called **scirrhous carcinoma** (due to the increased fibrous tissue stroma).
- The connective tissue is responsible for dimpling of the skin and retraction of the nipple.

Medullary carcinoma and mucinoid carcinoma are encapsulated cancers that usually occur combined with another form of cancer.

Paget's disease is an abnormality of the nipple usually associated with an underlying cancer (usually ductal carcinoma).

Inflammatory carcinoma is a very aggressive form of breast cancer characterized by rapid enlargement of the breast and is associated with erythema, warmth, pain, and involvement of the subdermal lymphatics.

Staging of Breast Cancer

- Staging of breast cancer is important for the choice of therapy and to determine patient prognosis.
- The TNM classification is used to stage breast cancer and is shown in the following table.

Stage	Histology	Tumor size T	Node involvement N	Distal metastasis M	10-year survival rate
Stage 0	Noninvasive	Any	—	—	—
Stage I	Invasive	< 2 cm			
Stage II		2-5 cm <5 cm	Negative	Negative	70-90%
	Invasive	>5 cm	Negative Positive	Negative	50-70%
Stage III		> 5cm	Negative		
	Invasive	skin or cell			
Stage IV		wall invasion	Positive or Negative	Negative	20-50%
		Any			
			Positive or Negative	Positive	Poor

CANCERS IN ORDER OF PROGNOSIS

1. LCIS and DCIS
2. Paget's disease
3. Well-differentiated adenocarcinoma
4. Medullary carcinoma
5. Colloid or mucinoid CA
6. Tubular CA
7. Infiltrating ductal/lobular CA
8. Inflammatory CA

Increasing Malignancy

- If a breast cancer spreads, it most commonly metastasizes to the lymph nodes.
- Common sites of distant metastasis include the **lungs, liver, bones, and brain**.

Treatment Options for Breast Cancer

- Surgery is the form of treatment for most cancers at an early stage (I or II).
- Chemotherapy, hormonal therapy, and radiotherapy along with surgery are recommended for more advanced disease (stage III and IV). The role of surgery in advanced disease is primarily palliation. Surgical options include:

Radical mastectomy

- Radical mastectomy is essentially obsolete
- Radical mastectomy involves the removal of all breast, pectoralis muscles, and axillary contents.

Modified radical mastectomy

- Modified radical mastectomy is the most commonly applied treatment.
- Modified radical mastectomy involves the removal of all breast and axillary contents without pectoralis muscles.
- Modified radical mastectomy has the same survival benefit as radical mastectomy.

Breast conservation therapy (BCT)

- BCT includes **segmental mastectomy**, **quadrantectomy**, or **lumpectomy**, which differ primarily by the amount of breast tissue removed.
- BCT consists of removal of the breast tumor with negative margins, axillary dissection, and breast irradiation.
- These procedures have the same survival benefit as radical mastectomy.
- Some contraindications include patients whose cancers cannot be excised without negative margins, patients who cannot receive radiation therapy, multicentric tumors, large tumor size, and tumors associated with extensive intraductal disease.

Patients with more advanced disease may benefit from additional treatment.

Chemotherapy is indicated for patients with a high probability of harboring micrometastases. These include patients with stage II and III disease. Any patient with positive nodes should receive chemotherapy.

Hormonal manipulations

- Generally is only considered for estrogen- or progesterone-sensitive tumors
- Tamoxifen is an estrogen antagonist that can be used as an adjuvant treatment in postmenopausal patients with estrogen-binding tumors.

- Premenopausal women may undergo bilateral oophorectomy to remove the endogenous source of estrogen (ablative surgery).

Radiation Therapy is used to control local disease after breast conservation therapy and may be used as a palliative treatment for specific metastases.

Treatment of metastasis may be done with:

- Chemotherapy
- Radiation therapy as a palliative treatment for specific metastases
- Hormonal manipulations such as tamoxifen or ablative surgery.

6 | UROLOGY

Renal Masses

General
- Renal masses can be benign or malignant.
- **Over 70% of renal masses are benign and cystic in nature.**
- The most common primary tumor is renal cell carcinoma (**RCC**).
- Transitional cell carcinoma is another type of cancer that may originate from the renal pelvis.
- RCC commonly metastasizes to bone, lungs and brain.
  - Metastasis may also occur to the contralateral kidney and liver.
- Other types of kidney tumors include: sarcoma, adenoma, and oncocytoma.

Clinical Manifestations
- Cystic masses are usually asymptomatic
- Hematuria is the most common symptom of renal cancer
- Renal masses rarely present with:
  - Palpable mass
  - Weight loss and anemia
  - Hypertension

Diagnosis
- History and physical examination
- Urinalysis
- Intravenous pyelogram (IVP)

- Ultrasound
- If a mass is suspected with the above studies, a CT-scan of the kidneys should be performed with IV contrast.
- Metastatic workup includes:
  - Chest x-ray
  - LFTs
  - Abdominal CT-scan

Management

- The management of a nonmetastatic solid mass is radical nephrectomy.
- Surgery includes:
  - Nephrectomy
  - Excision of the adrenal gland
  - Excision of Gerota's fascia
- The prognosis of RCC depends on the stage of the cancer.

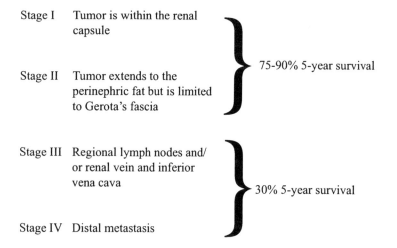

Stage I	Tumor is within the renal capsule	
Stage II	Tumor extends to the perinephric fat but is limited to Gerota's fascia	75-90% 5-year survival
Stage III	Regional lymph nodes and/ or renal vein and inferior vena cava	30% 5-year survival
Stage IV	Distal metastasis	

Prostate

General

- The prostate is an exocrine gland whose function is the production a minor fraction of the ejaculate.
- The weight of a normal prostate is about 20 gm.
- Pathologically the prostate is divided into three zones:

- The different disorders of the prostate can grouped into three categories:

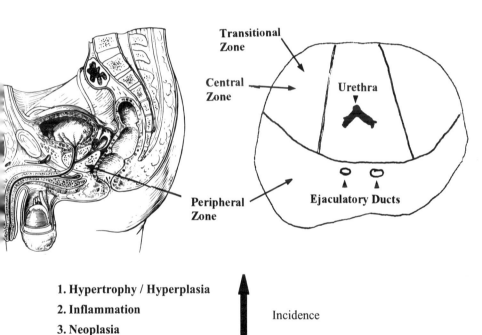

1. **Hypertrophy / Hyperplasia**
2. **Inflammation**
3. **Neoplasia**

Incidence

Hypertrophy/Hyperplasia

General

- Benign prostatic hypertrophy (**BPH**) is the most common condition affecting the prostate.
- BPH is a condition that involves both hyperplasia ($\uparrow$ cell #) and hypertrophy ($\uparrow$ size) of the prostate.
- The prostate is exquisitely responsive to dihydrotestosterone (DHT) for its growth.

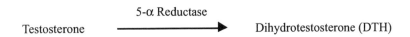

Testosterone $\xrightarrow{\text{5-}\alpha\text{ Reductase}}$ Dihydrotestosterone (DTH)

- The prostate begins to concentrate DHT at age 30. Hypertrophy and hyperplasia continues to occur. Hypertrophy and hyperplasia can be observed in 90% of individuals at age 80.
- Enlargement occurs primarily in the transition zone of the prostate.
- BPH does NOT lead to an increased risk of prostatitis or cancer.

Clinical Manifestations
- The clinical manifestations of BPH are primarily due to obstruction caused by hypertrophy and hyperplasia of the transitional zone of the prostate.
  - ↓ urinary stream
  - hesitancy
  - frequency
  - dribbling
  - retention
  - nocturia
  - urgency

Diagnosis
- History and physical examination
- Digital rectal exam reveals a smooth, soft, enlarged prostate which may or may not be asymmetric.
- BPH produces no urinalysis abnormalities.
- Flow rate analysis reveals decreased urinary stream.
- Catheterization or ultrasound post-void residual. Ultrasound may reveal hydronephrosis.
- Intravenous pyelography (IVP) may reveal thickening of the detrusor or "J-hooking" of the ureters.

Treatment

Medical Treatment

- α_1-adrenergic blockers (e.g., doxazosin, terazosin) provide symptomatic relief by relaxing smooth muscle cells in the prostate and bladder neck.
- 5-α-reductase inhibitors (e.g., finasteride) inhibits the conversion of testosterone to the active form, dihydrotestosterone. This decreases androgenic activity to the prostate cells and causes a 50% decrease in prostate size in six months.

Surgical Treatment

- Open prostatectomy is recommended for large prostates (> 80 gm).
- Transurethral prostatectomy (TURP):
  - Obstructing prostatic tissue is removed by electrocautery under direct visualization.
  - This is the most common operation performed to relieve the symptoms of BPH.
- Transurethral incision of the prostate (TUIP):
  - Incision of the prostate relieves obstruction for smaller prostates (< 20 gm).
- Other surgical treatments under investigation include thermotherapy and laser therapy.

Inflammation

General

- Prostatitis can be caused by one or more of the following conditions:
  - Acute bacterial prostatitis (ABP)
  - Chronic bacterial prostatitis (CBP)
  - Chronic nonbacterial prostatitis (CNBP)
- Acute prostatitis is most commonly caused by retrograde migration of Gram-negative rods (most commonly *E. coli*) to the prostate. Chronic bacterial prostatitis is caused by repeated infections of the prostate. The etiology of nonbacterial prostatitis is less clear and may be related to spasms of the pelvic floor muculature.

Clinical Manifestations

- ABP presents with common signs of infection:
  - Fever

- Chills
- Dysuria

- CBP may present as recurrent UTIs.
- Prostatitis may present with signs and symptoms of obstruction similar to BPH.
- The hallmark of prostatitis is pain.
    - ABP and CBP may present with dysuria, abdominal pain, painful ejaculation or perineal discomfort.
    - NBCP usually causes abdominal pain or perineal discomfort.

Diagnosis

- History and physical examination
    - Patients with ABP present with fever and chills and have and exquisitely tender prostate. These patients should only have a brief gentle prostate examination to confirm the diagnosis. Prostate massage should not be performed.
    - Patients with CBP usually have a protracted recurring problem and typically do not have fever or chills.
    - Rectal exam reveals tenderness.
    - Expressed prostatic secretion (EPS) is obtained by gentle massage of the prostate during a rectal exam.
    - If EPS > 15 WBC/HPF = Prostatitis
    - If culture → growth = Bacterial prostatitis.

Treatment

- ABP is treated with IV broad-spectrum antibiotics
- CBP and CNBP are treated symptomatically with oral antibiotics (usually quinolones), NSAIDs, sitz baths, stool softeners, and close follow-up.
    - ↑ fluid intake and ↓alcohol consumption are recommended prophylactic measures.

Prostate Neoplasm

General

- Prostate cancer is the most common cancer and the second leading cause of death due to malignancy in men.
- The majority of cases of prostate cancer originate in the peripheral zone of the prostate.
- Prostate cancer is graded by the **Gleason** grading system. This system establishes the degree of differentiation of tumor cells. The higher the grade given to

the specimen the more the degree of de-differentiation and the poorer the outcome.

- Prostate cancer is staged according to the degree of local and distal invasion:

TNM
Stage

- **Stage A** - microscopic, clinically unsuspected tumors found
  at the time of TURP.
  - **A1** - well-differentiated tumors with three or fewer foci .... **TI A**
  - **A2** - poorly-differentiated tumors with more than
          three foci .... **TI B**
  - **Stage B-** tumors confined to the prostate **T2**
  - **Stage C**-cancers that have spread beyond the prostatic
      capsule into the pelvis, but not to distant sites. **T3**
- **Stage D**-tumors that have spread to distant sites- usually bone (50% of new cases).
- **TIC** are tumors with normal DRE. They are discovered because an elevated prostate-specific antigen (PSA).

Clinical Manifestations

- Most patients diagnosed with prostate cancer are asymptomatic and the cancer is discovered due to an elevated PSA.
- Prostate cancer may also present with BPH-like symptoms. Prostate cancer must be ruled out with a DRE and PSA in any man presenting with BPH symptoms.
- Patients with metastatic bone disease present with bone pain in the low back and hips, as well as weight loss.

Diagnosis

- History and physical examination
  - Digital rectal examination
- Transrectal ultrasonography (**TRUS**) is used to direct the needle for prostate biopsies.
- Prostate-specific antigen (**PSA**):
  - Serine protease that is produced by normal and neoplastic epithelial cells.
  - PSA may be elevated in:
    - BPH
    - Prostatititis
    - Neoplasm
  - PSA > 10 → 66% chance biopsy shows cancer

- PSA = 4-10 → 22% chance biopsy shows cancer
- Elevated PSA is useful to detect prostate cancer (prior to surgery) and recurrence after surgery.

Treatment

- Patients with at least a 10-year life expectancy should undergo removal of the prostate. Curative therapy is considered with these patients and includes:
  - Radical prostatectomy performed via a perineal approach or a retropubic route.
    - Entire prostate, prostatic capsule, seminal vesicles, ampullary portion of the ductus deferens, and pelvic lymph nodes are removed.
- In patients with metastatic disease (Stage D), treatment consists of hormonal therapy:
  - Bilateral orchiectomy
  - LH-RH analog (e.g., leuprolide) suppress testosterone to the castrated range. This drug will cause hot flashes, fatigue and weight gain.
  - Antiandrogens (e.g., flutamide) may be used in conjunction with LH-RH analogs. Side effects include gynecomastia and GI disturbances.
- Chemotherapy is not effective in the treatment of stage D disease.
- Patients with stage D disease have an average survival of 3 years.

Urinary Bladder

General
- The various disorders affecting the bladder can be grouped into the following categories:

  - Congenital
  - Inflammatory
  - Traumatic
  - Degenerative
  - Malignant

Congenital
- The most common congenital problem affecting the bladder is vesicouretral reflux (VUR).
- VUR occurs due to poor development of the distal ureter resulting in reflux of urine.
- VUR is classified into five grades depending on the degree of reflux.

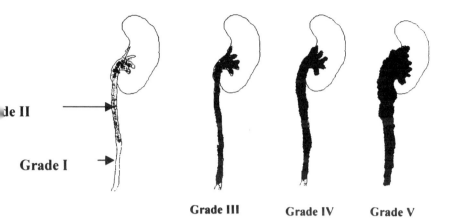

Clinical Manifestations
- VUR is usually seen in children who present with recurrent UTIs.

Diagnosis
- The diagnosis is made by voiding cystourethrogram (VCUG) in which contrast media is injected into the bladder followed by radiography.

Treatment
- Grade I/II VUR usually resolves with age.
    - Antibiotic prophylaxis should be provided to protect the kidney from infection
    - Children should be closely followed up with urine cultures.
- Grade III-V should be treated with surgery.
    - Ureteral reimplantation

Inflammatory
- Bacterial cystitis and interstitial cystitis are the most common inflammatory processes affecting the bladder.

Bacterial Cystitis

General
- Bacterial cystitis is more common in females.
- In males, it may be due to incomplete emptying of the bladder.
- The most common bacteria causing bacterial cystitis are Gram-negative rods in the Enterobacteriaceae family.
- 80% of UTIs are caused by *E. coli.*

Clinical Manifestations
- Dysuria
- Frequency
- Urgency
- Nocturia
- Hematuria
- +/- fever

Diagnosis
- History and physical examination
- Urinalysis (clean catch)
- Urine culture

Treatment
- Antibiotic treatment should be empiric when the diagnosis is suspected.
- Empiric treatment should be followed by specific antibiotic treatment based on culture and sensitivity results from a clean catch urine specimen.

Interstitial cystitis

General
- Interstitial cystitis is more commonly seen in females.
- It is of unknown etiology.
- The bladder is chronically inflamed and may become fibrotic.

Clinical Manifestations
- Suprapubic pain related to urination
- Urinary frequency and urgency
- Symptoms wax and wane

Diagnosis
* Interstitial cystitis is a diagnosis of exclusion.
* Bladder tumor and UTI should be ruled out.

Treatment
* Temporary symptomatic treatment may include bladder dilatation and installation of anti-inflammatory agents such as dimethyl sulfoxide (DMSO).

Trauma

General
* Trauma to the bladder may be the result of penetrating trauma (e.g., gun shot wounds, stab wounds, and instrumentation) or blunt trauma (e.g., motor vehicle accidents).

Clinical Presentation
* Severe suprapubic pain
* Inability to void
* Hematuria
* Most commonly the clinical presentation is due to blunt trauma and is often associated with pelvic fracture.

Diagnosis
* History and physical examination
* Cystogram in the emergency room should be performed to rule out bladder rupture and assess if the rupture is intra- or extraperitoneal.

Treatment
* Small extraperitoneal ruptures to the bladder resolve spontaneously in two weeks with a Foley catheter drainage.
* Large injuries to the bladder and intraperitoneal bladder ruptures require surgical repair.

Urinary Incontinence

Types of incontinence
* **Stress incontinence** – urinary leakage following an increase in intra-abdominal pressure (e.g., during coughing, laughing, sneezing).
   - This is common in older women with history of multiple vaginal deliveries.

- **Urge incontinence** – urinary leakage immediately following a sensation of urinary urgency.
    - Results from involuntary muscle contractions.
    - This is common in older men and women.
- **Overflow incontinence** – ongoing leakage of small volumes of urine that typically occurs in patients with urinary retention.

Diagnosis
- History and physical examination
    - General medical conditions
    - Pattern of voiding
    - Voiding record
- Laboratory studies
    - Urinalysis
    - Urine culture
    - Cytology
- Postvoid residual (PVR) measurement (catheterization of patient after voiding)
    - Residual volume greater than 100mL suggests bladder weakness or obstruction.

Treatment
- Treatment is dictated by the type of incontinence.

Stress incontinence
- Kegel's exercises - patient practices interrupting voiding; 20 contractions 4 times a day.
- Surgery to restore the anatomic position of the bladder neck and urethra (e.g., bladder neck suspensions and urethral sling procedures).

Urge incontinence
- Anticholinergic agents and tricyclic antidepressants (e.g., imipramine) decrease muscle contractility.

Overflow incontinence
- α-adrenergic antagonists (e.g., doxazosin, terazosin) decrease bladder obstruction from BPH.
- Relief of obstruction (e.g., BPH) with surgery (e.g., TURP).
- If there is an atonic bladder and no outlet obstruction, clean intermittent self-catheterization will provide relief.

Malignancy

Bladder Carcinoma

General

- Bladder cancer is the fourth most common cancer in males and eighth most common cancer in females.
- It is two to three times more common in men.
- 85% are transitional cell carcinomas.
- Risk factors include:
    - Exposure to aromatic amines used in the synthesis of dyes
    - Smoking
    - Recurrent UTIs.
    - Employment
        - Truck drivers
        - Painters
        - Workers in textile and paper manufacturing

Clinical presentation

- Hematuria
- Dysuria
- Frequency
- Urgency
- Weight loss and bone pain in advanced disease

Diagnosis

- History and physical examination
- Intravenous pyelography (ureteral obstruction, hydronephrosis, filling defects)
- Urinary cytology
- Cystoscopy

Staging	Jewett-Strong-Marshall classification	TNM
Invades mucosa	O	Ta
Invades submucosa	A	T1
Invades muscularis	B1	T2
Extends into perivesical fat	C	T3
Metastatic	D	T4

Treatment
- Superficial Cancer
  - Transurethral resection
- Recurrence may be prevented with intravesicular therapy:
  - Mitomycin
  - Thiotepa
  - Bacillus Calmette-Guérin (BCG)
- Invasive disease:
  - Radical cystectomy involves removal of the prostate and seminal vesicles in males and uterus, fallopian tubes, and ovaries in females.
  - Radiation
  - Chemotherapy and radiation
- Metastatic disease
  - Chemotherapy:
    - cisplatin
    - methotrexate
    - doxorubicin
    - cyclophosphamide, and/or vinblastine
- Most patients with metastatic disease die within 2 years.

Urolithiasis

General
- Urinary calculi may be caused by urine supersaturated with calcium oxalate or uric acid, causing crystallization.
- If the crystals are trapped, they form stones.
- Formation of stones may lead to obstruction.
- Common sites of obstruction are the ureteropelvic junction, ureterovesicular junction, and the intersection of the ureter and the iliac vessels.

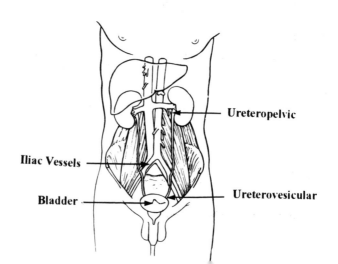

• The different types of stones are shown in the table below:

Type of stone	Characteristics	Predisposing Factors
Calcium oxalate	· 75% of all stones · Radiopaque (can be seen by x-ray)	· Diet ↑ Ca^{++} · Hyperparathyrodism · Warm climate · Family history of RTA type I · Drugs:triamterene, acetazolamide · IBD
Struvite	· 15% of all stones · It is composed of Mg-NH_4-PO_4 · It is associated with infections · Causes ≤ urine pH > 7.2 · Large stones described as staghorns	· Urea-splitting bacterial UTIs · Urinary obstruction
Uric acid	· 7% of all stones · Radiolucent	· Diet: ↑ purine intake · History of gout · Hyperuricosuria
Cystine	· 1% of all stones	Family history

Clinical Manifestations

• Patients with symptomatic urinary stones present with acute onset of severe flank pain radiating to the groin, often accompanied by nausea and vomiting, which results from urinary obstruction.

• Patients may also present with frequency and urgency.

• Asymptomatic stones may present with hematuria as the only sign.

Evaluation

• History and physical examination should provide information on diet, history of hyperparathyroidism, and costovertebral angle tenderness.

• Laboratory

  • Urinalysis and urinary culture: hematuria, WBCs, RBCs, urinary pH (RTA).

  • CBC with differential and electrolytes with creatinine: ″WBC, ″BUN/Cr ratio,

  • Serum Ca^{++} and PTH

  • Kidney-ureters-bladder (KUB) plain film: 80% of calculi can be detected by plain films of the abdomen.

Radiodensities:

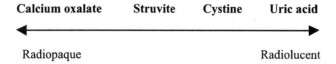

Diagnosis

- The diagnosis is made by KUB or intravenous pyelogram (IVP)— contrast material in injected IV, which collects in the urinary system and an x-ray of the abdomen is taken.

Management

- Hydration
- Pain control
- Combination of obstructing stone and fever is a surgical emergency requiring drainage of pus in kidney with either ureteral stent or percutaneous nephrostomy tube.

Treatment is largely dependent on the type, size, and location of the stone.

- **Calcium oxalate stones**
    - These stones do not respond well to medical therapy (e.g., hydration or alkalization of the urine).
    - If the stone is located in the kidney, extracorporeal shock wave lithotripsy (ESWL) is appropriate.
    - ESWL consists of the transmission of a focused shock wave from outside of the body to the calculus, causing the stone to fragment.
    - Renal stones < 5mm usually pass spontaneously.
    - Following formation of the first stone, patients should be advised to increase fluid intake.
    - Underlying disease causing hypercalcemia (e.g., hyperparathyroidism) should be treated.

- **Struvite stones** should be treated with management of the underlying infection.
    - Often, larger stones require percutaneous endoscopy and removal.

- **Uric acid stones**
    - Urine alkalization and aggressive hydration may dissolve the stone.

- Patients should be advised to decrease animal protein intake, and maintain alkaline urine.
- Allopurinol is used for prophylaxis.

- **Cysteine stones** do not respond well to ESWL.
  - Treatment consists of urine alkalization or administration of α-mercaptopropionylglycine.
  - Patients should be advised to decrease meat intake, increase water intake, and maintain a high urinary pH.

7 | OTOLARYNGOLOGY

Neck Masses

General
The wide variety of neck masses can be grouped into three categories: Congenital, Inflammatory, and Neoplastic.

Clinical Manifestations
- The clinical manifestations of a neck mass depend on the category the mass falls into:

	Congenital	Inflammatory	Neoplastic
• Age of onset	birth-young adult	child-young adult	child-adult
• Type of onset	persistently present	recent, short duration	chronic onset, slow growth
• Characteristic of mass	soft, painless	soft, tender	firm,solid, fixed
• Symptoms	stridor, dyspnea, dysphagia	fever, pain/ tenderness erythema	weight loss, stridor, dyspnea, dysphagia, +/- pain
• Predisposing factors	-	previous upper respiratory tract infection	alcohol, tobacco

- **Congenital masses**:
  - These are characteristically soft, painless, persistent, and occur early in life.
  - Location and characteristics can distinguish the various types of congenital masses commonly encountered.

- The following are common congenital masses:
    1. Dermoid Cyst (DC)
        - Dermoid cysts occur due to a defect in the fusion of somatic segments.
        - Accumulation of sebaceous secretions lead to swelling.
        - **These masses usually occur in the midline of the neck.**
    2. Thyroglossal duct cyst (TDC)
        - These occur due to remnants of the thyroid gland during its migration from the base of the tongue (foramen cecum) to its adult position.
        - Functioning thyroid epithelium leads to swelling from the accumulation of fluid.
        - **These masses also occur in the midline of the neck and move up and down with swallowing.**
    3. Pharyngeal cleft cyst (PCC)
        - Branchial Cysts are remnants of pharyngeal clefts.
        - **These masses usually occur in the anteriolateral aspect of the neck.**
    4. Cystic hygroma (CH)
        - Cystic Hygromas occur when there is obliteration of lymphatic drainage.
        - These masses are present at the time of birth.
        - **These masses are frequently located in the posterior aspect of the sternocleidomastoid muscle.**

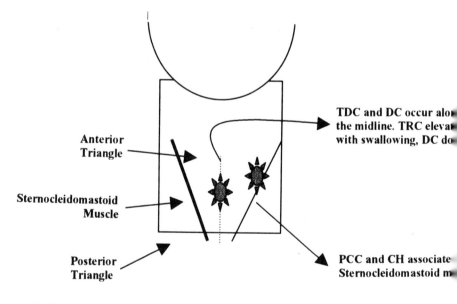

Anterior Triangle

Sternocleidomastoid Muscle

Posterior Triangle

TDC and DC occur alon the midline. TRC elevat with swallowing, DC do

PCC and CH associate Sternocleidomastoid m

- **Inflammatory masses:**
    - This is the most common type of neck mass affecting children and young adults. Symptoms of infection such as fever, pain/tenderness, and erythema are common characteristics of these masses.
    - Common inflammatory masses are the result of an infectious agent, typically in the salivary glands or lymph nodes:

1. Viral
   - Viral lymphadenitis
2. Bacterial
   - Bacterial adenitis
   - Ludwig's angina (bacterial infection that results from dental infections)
3. Fungal
   - Fungal adenitis (occurs in the immunocompromised patient)

- **Neoplastic masses**
  - A progressively enlarging, firm, solid mass in the adult patient should be considered cancer unless proven otherwise.
  - Neoplastic masses can be benign or malignant. The most common benign masses occurring in the neck include lipomas and neurogenic tumors.
  - Lymphoma is the most common malignant neoplasm in children and young adults. In the adult population with history of alcohol and tobacco use, the most common type of malignancy is metastatic squamous cell carcinoma.
  - The most common midline tumor in both children and adults originates in the thyroid gland.
  - Benign thyroid masses include Graves' disease and toxic thyroiditis.

- **Malignancies of the thyroid gland**

  Malignancies of the thyroid arise from three different origins:

  1. Follicular cells
     A. *Papillary carcinoma* is the most common type of thyroid CA. It is characterized by slow growth and carries a good prognosis.
     B. *Follicular carcinoma* is more aggressive than papillary CA and can be differentiated by its capsular and vascular invasion. This type of cancer concentrates thyroid hormone readily.
     C. *Anaplastic carcinoma* also originates from follicular cells, but the cells have become dedifferentiated. Hence, this CA carries the poorest prognosis of all thyroid CAs.

  2. C-cells
     A. *Medullary* carcinoma is often genetically transmitted and is associated with the multiple endocrine neoplasm syndrome (MEN syndrome). This cancer also carries a poor prognosis. MEN syndromes include:

MEN I	MEN IIa	MEN IIb
· Parathyroid hyperplasia	· Medullary carcinoma	· Medullary carcinoma
· Pituitary adenoma	· Parathyroid hyperplasia	· Pheochromocytoma
· Pancreatic tumors	· Pheochromocytoma	· Mucosal neuromas
		· Marfanoid habitus

  3. Lymphoid tissue
     A. Lymphoma

Diagnosis

- History and physical examination are particularly rewarding in the evaluation of a neck mass.

- Flexible fiberoptic examination should be used to evaluate laryngeal/esophageal involvement.

- Ultrasound is useful in establishing the cystic or solid nature of a neck mass.

- CT is indicated if the nature of the mass is uncertain. CT should also be considered in patients with metastatic squamous cell carcinoma to evaluate the degree of metastasis and the amount of involvement of the primary tumor.

- Fine-needle aspiration (FNA) can in most cases establish a definitive diagnosis of a neck mass.

- Biopsy should not be performed in a neck mass which is suspected of being a metastatic carcinoma. Instead, work-up should be done to locate a primary tumor. This includes:

  - Complete head and neck examination
  - Chest x-ray
  - CT or MRI
  - Triple endoscopy (direct laryngoscopy, esophagoscopy, bronchoscopy)

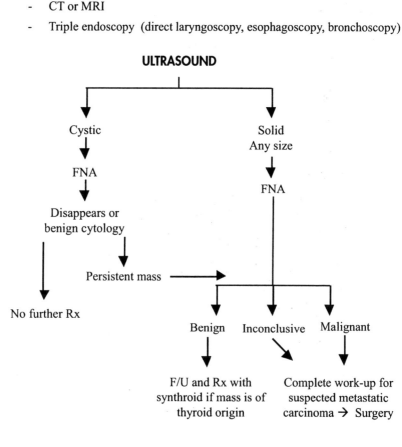

Management
- **Congenital Masses**

Thyroglossal duct cyst
Dermoid cyst
Pharyngeal cleft cyst
Cystic hygroma

} Surgical removal is indicated for the management of these neck masses. TDC should be treated by removal of the cyst trunk and hyoid bone at the midpoint to avoid recurrence (Sistrunk procedure).

- **Inflammatory masses:**

Viral → is a self-limiting condition. Thus, supportive management is usually the only indication.
Bacterial → appropriate antibiotic coverage. Surgical debridement may be indicated if the mass or infection persists.
Fungal → amphotericin B and surgical debridement.

- **Neoplastic masses:**

  - Benign masses require surgical excision.

  - Malignant neoplasms require radiation, surgery, or both. Radiation therapy should be directed at the primary tumor site. Radical or modified neck dissection should follow radiation therapy depending on the size of the tumor.

- **Thyroid masses:**

  - Surgery is the treatment of choice for thyroid cancer. Surgical options for the management of thyroid cancer include:
    - Total thyroidectomy
    - Subtotal thyroidectomy
    - Lobectomy and removal of the isthmus

  - The type of surgery performed depends on the type and size of the tumor and the surgeon performing the operation.

  - Other treatment options include treatment with iodine 131 (I^{131}) for those cancers that concentrate iodine (papillary and follicular carcinoma).

- An alternative approach to neck masses is an anatomic one. The following table summarizes neck masses by anatomic location.

Triangles of the Neck

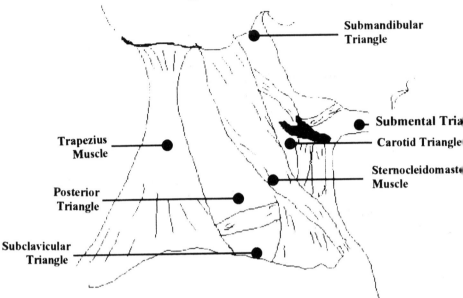

Submandibular Triangle

Submental Tria

Carotid Triangle

Sternocleidomaste Muscle

Trapezius Muscle

Posterior Triangle

Subclavicular Triangle

Anatomic Location of Masses of the Neck

Midline of the Neck	Posterior Triangle	Submandibular Triangle	Submental Triangle
1. Thyroid mass	1. Pharyngeal cleft cyst	1. Inflammatory	1. Inflammatory
2. Thyroglossal duct cyst	2. Cystic hygroma	2. Infectious (e.g., salivary glands)	2. Infectious (e.g., lymphadenopathy)
3. Dermoid cyst	3. Lymphadenopathy	3. Neoplastic	3. Neoplastic
4. Neoplastic	4. Neoplastic		

8 | ORTHOPEDIC SURGERY

> • Fractures are breaks in the bone or loss of
> continuity anywhere along the bones.
>
> • A subluxation is a partial loss of contact
> at joint surfaces.
>
> • A dislocation is complete loss of contact at
> joint surfaces.

Common Fractures:

General
• Fractures are broadly categorized into two groups:
  - **Closed Fractures** are fractures in which the skin remains intact.
  - **Open Fractures** are fractures in which there is communication of the
    bone with the external environment.
    - This includes pelvic fractures that may communicate with the rectum or
      vagina and are not readily visible by rapid inspection.
    - Open fractures are contaminated and mandate aggressive treatment. Open
      fractures are further classified into grades:

OPEN FRACTURE GRADES

- **Grade I**   < 1 cm skin laceration
- **Grade II**   > 1 cm < 10 cm skin laceration
- **Grade IIIa** Massive tissue loss
- **Grade IIIb** Tissue loss and extensive contamination
- **Grade IIIc** Major vascular injury has occurred

Common Fractures

- **Greenstick Fracture** is a fracture that is incomplete. Only one side of the bone (one cortex) is disrupted.
- **Stress Fracture** is a fracture caused by repeated stress on a bone.
- **Pathologic Fracture** is a fracture that occurs in a diseased bone (e.g., osteoporotic bone).
- **Simple Fracture** is a fracture that generates at the most two bone fragments.
- **Comminuted Fracture** is fracture that leads to more than two bone fragments.

Fractures involving the growth plate

- Fractures involving the growth plate are categorized using the **Salter-Harris classification**:
  - **Type I** fracture occurs when there is separation of the epiphysis from the metaphysis. There is no longitudinal disruption of either the epiphysis or the metaphysis.
  - **Type II** fracture consists of epiphysis-metaphysis separation and fracture of the metaphysis.
  - **Type III** fracture is an intra-articular fracture as it involves the epiphysis.
  - **Type IV** fracture involves epiphysis-metaphysis separation and longitudinal fracture involving both the metaphysis and diaphysis. This is also an intra-articular type of fracture.
  - **Type V** fracture is a fracture that involves crushing of the epiphyseal plate.
- All growth plate fractures have the potential to cause growth disturbances. The higher the grade, the greater the risk of growth abnormalities.

Clinical Manifestations

- Most fractures occur as a result of trauma and present with complaints of recent injury.
- Symptoms of fracture include pain, swelling, and deformity.
- Physical examination reveals tenderness, deformity, swelling, and +/- erythema.
- Fractures involving the vasculature may present with decreased or absent pulses and hemodynamic manifestations.
- Fractures with nerve injury may present with sensory or motor deficits.

Diagnosis

- History and physical examination
- Appropriate x-rays
- Bone scan, CT and MRI are seldom needed to establish the diagnosis.

Management

- ABCs should be assessed in a patient presenting with a fracture. This will also allow the examiner to establish the degree of vascular and/or nervous involvement.

- All fractures should be splinted as soon as possible after assessment of ABCs.

- Reduction means restoration of bone alignment.

- There are two types of reduction procedures that can be performed:

    - **Closed reduction** is bone aligment by manipulation without surgical exposure.

    - **Open reduction** is bone aligment performed by surgical exposure. An open fracture should be managed by open reduction.

- Maintenance of alignment:

    - There are various methods that can be used for maintenance of the reduction.

    ```
    1. Casting
    2. Traction
    3. Internal fixation
    4. External fixation
    ```

- All open fractures are contaminated by definition and require immediate intervention:

    - IV antibiotics should be quickly started with Gram-positive coverage for grade I fractures and Gram-positive plus anaerobic coverage for greater than grade II fractures.

    - Tetanus prophylaxis

    - Surgical debridement

    - Lavage should be rapidly performed to avoid extension of the infection.

    - Open reduction and internal fixation (ORIF).

- Other indications for open reduction include:

    - Inrta-articular fractures (including Salter-Harris fractures type III-V)

    - Close reduction failure

    - Vascular/neural involvement

Orthopedic Emergencies

- Orthopedic emergencies include:

> 1. Open fractures
> 2. Compartment syndrome
> 3. Fractures with vascular/neural involvement
> 4. Bone/articular infections (osteomyelitis/septic arthritis)
> 5. Hip fractures

Compartment syndrome

General
- Compartment syndrome is the drastic increase in pressure of muscle groups, which are normally enclosed in osseo-fascial compartments.
- Common causes of compartment syndrome include:
    - Fractures
    - Muscle contusions
    - Crush injuries
- Compartment pressure may be so elevated such that muscle necrosis may ensue.
- The following are fractures that commonly lead to compartment syndromes:
    - Proximal third of the tibia
    - Supracondylar humerus
    - Radius and ulnar fractures occurring concomitantly

Clinical Manifestations
- Signs and symptoms of the compartment syndrome:

    - Pain
    - Paresthesia
    - Pallor
    - Paralysis

- **Pulses** may be **present** even in severe cases of compartment syndrome and should not be considered as a clinical manifestation of the compartment syndrome.

Diagnosis

- History and physical examination
- Compartment systolic pressure > 30 mm Hg
- High degree of suspicion is sufficient to initiate treatment

Treatment

- Treatment consists of immediate decompression by open fasciotomy.

9 | NEUROSURGERY

Head Trauma

General

- Acute head trauma represents a dangerous, but often treatable, condition requiring prompt diagnosis and treatment.
- Of particular concern in the case of head trauma are:
    - injury to the brain itself
    - intracranial hematomas, and either open or closed skull fractures
- In many cases, a great part of the danger to the brain is the result of increased intracranial pressure.
- Small increases in intracranial pressure are usually compensated for, but as the pressure rises to dangerous levels, there will be compression and displacement of intracranial structures.
- In order for cerebral perfusion to prevent brain ischemia, the mean systemic blood pressure should be at least 45 mm Hg greater than the intracranial pressure.
    - Normal ICP is 5-15 mm H_2O
    - ICP over 20 mm H_2O requires intervention.
- In addition to affecting cerebral perfusion, elevated intracranial pressure may also exert a mass effect on the brain.
    - **Transtentorial herniation**, in which the brain stem is displaced through the foramen magnum, is the most life-threatening event caused by elevated ICP.
    - Space occupying lesions such as local bleeds may also exert local pressures which result in **focal neurologic dysfunction**.

Clinical Manifestations

- Because of the potentially devastating effects of increased intracranial pressure, the symptoms must be recognized early and a diagnosis made.

- **Symptoms of elevated ICP include:**
  - Headache
  - Nausea
  - Vomiting
  - Double vision (diplopia)
- **Signs of elevated ICP include:**
  - Papilledema
  - Altered level of consciousness

Diagnosis and Evaluation of the Patient with Head Trauma

- Whenever possible, a history should be obtained to determine the nature of the injury and whether the patient's condition has deteriorated or improved since the time of the injury.
- The evaluation begins with the ABCs, which are often altered following head injury.
- Cushing's triad of physiologic respones to increased ICP:

---

1. Increased blood pressure
2. Bradycardia
3. Irregular respiration

- Once these basics have been stabilized, a neurological evaluation should be performed.

- **The neurological examination should assess :**
  - eye response
    - A unilateral, dilated, nonreactive pupil is suggestive of a focal mass lesion.
    - Bilateral fixed and dilated pupils suggest diffusely increased ICP.
    - If increased intracranial pressure is suspected, it should be treated as noted below and a CT-scan should be done to identify the cause.
  - verbal response
    - If the patient is poorly responsive, corneal and gag reflexes can be tested to evaluate brain stem function.
  - motor response

- The examination should also include checking for signs of cerebrospinal fluid leak (see skull fractures below).
- The head should then be inspected and palpated for lacerations or skull fractures.
- After taking cervical radiographs to rule out fractures or dislocations, skull films are taken to look for fractures and CSF leaks.

Eyes	Verbal	Motor
1. Not open	1. Makes no sounds	1. Does not move
2. Open to pain	2. Makes incomprehensible sounds	2. Decerebrate posture (arms in the extended posture)
3. Open to voice	3. Speaks inappropriate words	3. Decorticate posture (arms in the flexed posture)
4. Open spontaneously	4. Confused	4. Withdraws from pain
	5. Alert and oriented	5. Localizes painful stimulus
		6. Obeys commands

- A CT-scan of the head is needed for patients with potentially increased intracranial pressure, lateralizing neurological deficits, decreasing consciousness, poor response to commands, or significant headache.
  - CT-scans and MRI are helpful in making the diagnosis.

Treatment
- Medical management of increased intracranial pressure includes:
  - Elevating the patient's head to optimize venous drainage
  - Osmotic diuretics such as mannitol to cause a fluid shift out of the brain
  - Hyperventilation of the patient
  - Reversible sedation, pharmacologic paralysis
  - Pentobarbital coma as a last resort
- The surgical management of increased ICP is discussed below.

Epidural Hematoma

General
- An epidural hematoma is a collection of blood between the dura mater and the inner bony surface of the cranial cavity.
- Epidural hematomas are caused by tearing of the middle meningeal artery, often caused by bone fragments during skull fracture.

Clinical Manifestations
- These patients may have a period of consciousness which is followed by progressive headache, drowsiness, hemiparesis, and a dilated pupil on the side of the hemorrhage.
- Rapid onset of symptoms is the hallmark of epidural hematomas.

Diagnosis

- A CT-scan reveals the hematoma, which is commonly lens-shaped.
  - The outer and inner margins of the hematoma are usually smooth because the blood faces the smooth surface of the skull on one side and the dura on the other.

Treatment

- Once an epidural hematoma has been diagnosed, medical measures may be employed to delay further neurologic damage until an emergent craniotomy can be performed to remove the clot and prevent reaccumulation of the hematoma.

Subdural Hematoma

General

- A subdural hematoma is a hemorrage into the space between the brain and the dura mater.
- Subdural hematomas are caused by the tearing of the bridging veins between the cortical surface and the venous sinuses.
- Only minimal trauma is necessary to tear these veins, so subdural hematomas are more common than epidural hematomas.
- Subdural hematomas commonly occur in elderly patients who have fallen and in children who have been abused, especially by being shaken.

Clinical Manifestations

- The clinical manifestations of a subdural hematoma are more insidious than those for an epidural hematoma.
- Once symptoms present they are similar to those of an epidural hamatoma.

Diagnosis

- History and physical examination
- A CT-scan will commonly reveal a hematoma that has a smooth curved outline on the margin facing the dura and a grooved outline on the surface facing the brain.
- Subdural hematomas may be further identified because they generally do not cross the falx cerebri.

Treatment

- Subdural hematomas require prompt craniotomy with removal of the clot.

Basilar Skull Fracture

General

- Basilar skull fractures are often extensions of adjacent fractures but may occur independently due to forces on the floor of the middle cranial fossa or occiput.

Clinical Manifestations

- The four signs of a basilar skull fracture are:

> 1. Periorbital ecchymosis (**raccoon eyes**)
> 2. Ecchymosis over the mastoid process (**Battle's sign**)
> 3. **Hemotympanum** (blood behind the tympanic membrane)
> 4. **CSF leakage** in the form of rhinorrhea or otorrhea

- In the case of rhinorrhea, the CSF leak is through a disrupted cribriform plate.
- Other signs that may indicate basilar skull fracture include the loss of sense of smell, and loss of hearing and facial motion on one side.

Diagnosis

- History and physical examination
- CT-scan
- MRI

Treatment

- Patients with basilar skull ·fractures are not operated upon emergently, even if CSF leakage is evident, though they have the potential for further leakage and intracranial infection.
- Prophylactic antibiotics are often given and the patients are instructed to avoid maneuvers that increase intracranial pressure, such as coughing and changing head positions.
- If CSF leakage ceases after five days, the patient is permitted to walk.
- If leakage persists, lumbar spinal subarachnoid drainage may enhance healing.
- **Surgical closure** is sometimes required with leak localization by radionuclide or contrast CT-scanning.

Spinal Cord Trauma

General

- Approximately 10,000 patients per year in the United States become paraplegic or quadriplegic because of spinal cord injuries.

- **Vertical compression with flexion** is the main mechanism of injury in the thoracic spinal cord while extension or flexion is the main mechanism of injury in the cervical spinal cord.

Clinical Manifestations

- The immediate injury causes disruption of the capillaries with resulting local hemorrhages and edema.

- The early phases of injury are associated with ischemia secondary to swelling and vasoconstriction. Infarction of gray matter ensues and spreads both outward as well as rostrocaudally.

- Approximately eight hours after the injury there is global infarction at the level of injury. It is at this point that necrosis of the white matter and paralysis below the level of the lesion become irreversible.

- Cervical or high thoracic trauma regularly cause mild hypotension and bradycardia due to disruption of the sympathetic nervous system.

- Injuries above C5 cause quadriplegia and respirtory failure. The level of sensory loss helps determine the level of injury.

- Injuries at C5 and C6 result in weakened biceps while injuries at C4 and C5 result in weakened deltoids.

- C7 injuries cause weakness of the triceps and wrist extensors.

- Injuries at T1 and below cause paraplegia.

Evaluation and Treatment

- Any patient in whom a significant neck injury cannot be excluded should be placed in a sturdy cervical collar to prevent further injury to a potentially unstable spinal column.

- The patient's spinal alignment should be maintained from head to buttock.

- Blood pressure, respiratory status, and systemic injuries should be addressed and monitored.

- The neurologic examination of the patient focuses on neck or back pain, limb motion without moving the patient's head or body, trunk sensation, and deep tendon reflexes.

- Initial therapy is aimed at minimizing further injury by assuring respiratory and cardiovascular support.

- In cases of cervical spinal cord trauma, external traction is attempted to reduce spinal column displacement.

- Massive doses of steroids begun within eight hours of injury may minimize spinal cord paralysis.

- If x-rays suggest a fractured or dislocated vertebral body, surgical reduction should be undertaken rapidly.

- Many traumatic myelopathies have no associated fracture or dislocation. MRI is usually used to identify the site of the lesion so that surgical decompression may be performed.

- If the pathology is anterior, anterior decompression by vertebrectomy and/or discectomy is performed.

- If the pathology is posterior, decompression is performed from the back by laminectomy. Internal stabilization is then applied.

- The postsurgical care of patients with spinal cord injuries is best undertaken in specialized centers.

- Management consists of frequent bladder catheterization, monitoring the skin for ulcer formation, and physical rehabilitation. Over time, spasticity may develop, requiring medication, injections, or other interventions.

Cerebrovascular Disease

- Cerebrovascular disease may be caused by several pathologic processes involving the vasculature of the brain.

- The process may be intrinsic to the vessel (atherosclerosis), may originate remotely (an embolus from the heart), may be due to inadequate cerebral blood flow (an acute hypotensive episode), or may result from a ruptured blood vessel.

- A stroke is the sudden or rapid occurrence of neurologic dysfunction or loss of consciousness due to one of these processes. However, a number of conditions such as seizure, syncope, multiple sclerosis, and migraine may mimic a stroke.

- Risk factors for stroke include:

    - Hypertension
    - Smoking
    - Hypercholesterolemia
    - History of transient ischemic attacks (TIAs)
    - Atrial fibrillation
    - Drug abuse
    - Diabetes mellitus
    - Asymptomatic carotid bruits
    - Coagulopathies

Approximately 80 percent of strokes are due to ischemic cerebral infarction while 20 percent are due to brain hemorrhage.

- Ischemic strokes result from vascular obstruction or low perfusion states; hemorrhagic strokes result from vascular rupture.

- The chart below helps to differentiate between ischemic and hemorrhagic strokes:

	Ischemic Stroke	Hemorrhagic Stroke
Onset	Rapid (seconds)	Slower (minutes to hours)
Headache	Little or none	Present and often accompanied by nausea and vomiting
Consciousness	No change	Marked disturbance
Mortality rate	25%	70%

Ischemic Stroke

General
- Ischemic strokes may be divided into two broad categories:
  - Embolic
  - Thrombotic

- Embolic strokes tend to occur abruptly while thrombotic strokes are often heralded by transient symptoms, transient ischemic attacks (**TIA**), reversible ischemic neurological deficit (**RIND**), or a minor stroke.

- A transient ischemic attack is a cerebrovascular event with symptoms that completely resolve within 24 hours.

- The symptoms of a reversible ischemic neurological defect resolve after more than one day.

- The risk of having a completed stroke after having a TIA is approximately 5% per year.

- A history of sudden onset of neurological deficit establishes a working diagnosis of stroke.

- A physical examination should be performed to determine if there is a focal neurolgical deficit. In addition, the optic fundi should be visualized and the carotid and subclavian arteries auscultated. MRI, duplex sonography, and contrast angiography are all used to examine the cervical carotid arteries.

Treatment
- Carotid endarterectomy with medical therapy has been shown to decrease the future incidence of stroke over medical therapy alone. Carotid endarterectomy

is the treatment of choice for patients who have had a TIA, RIND, or minor stroke resulting from an arteriosclerotic lesion at the origin of the internal carotid artery which produces greater than 70% stenosis.

- Other treatment options, which may be used alone or in conjunction with endarterectomy, include anticoagulant (warfarin) and antiplatelet (aspirin) therapy.

Hypertensive Intracerebral Hemorrhage

General
- Hypertensive hemorrhage typically occurs in the basal ganglia.

- An artery arising from the middle cerebral artery, basilar artery, or circle of Willis is usually the source of the hemorrhage.

- The hemorrhage begins as a small mass and then spreads, growing in volume while displacing and compressing adjacent brain tissue.

- Edema in the compressed tissue often leads to an increasing mass effect and worsening clinical state.

- Hypertensive intracerebral hemorrhages are most common in patients with long-standing hypertension.

Clinical Manifestations
- These hemorrhages almost always occur while the patient is awake and usually evolve over a few minutes.

- Intracranial hemorrhage should be suspected in patients with a sudden severe headache (without a prior history of such headaches) or in a patient with a sudden change in consciousness.

- Nausea and vomiting often accompany these acute hemorrhages.

Diagnosis
- History and physical examination
- CT-scan can reliably detect acute hemorrhages greater than one centimeter in diameter.
- MRI, though very sensitive, is usually not necessary.
- Angiography may be used when the cause of the hemorrhage is uncertain.

Treatment
- Treatment of the hemorrhage depends upon its location.
- Patients with large lobar hematomas often benefit from hematoma evacuation by craniotomy.
- Evacuation of hematomas in deep structures such as the basal ganglia is more

controversial because of the potential for neurological deficits and the risks of surgery.

- Stereotaxic removal of these clots may have a role in treatment.

Subarachnoid Hemorrhage

General

- Aneurysms and arteriovenous malformations (AVMs) are the two most common causes of subarachnoid hemorrhage.

- Aneurysms most often occur at branch points of the major vessels at the base of the brain and are termed berry aneurysms.

- The most common location for such an aneurysm is in the anterior part of the circle of Willis.

Clinical Manifestations

- The clinical presentation of a subarachnoid hemorrhage is often described as a "thunderclap" headache, which has a sudden onset and is often described by patients as the **worst headache of their life**.

- The pain is typically worst at the onset and may improve slowly.

- The patient may also have neurologic deficits or an altered level of consciousness.

- Nausea, vomiting, and a stiff neck may also be present.

- Ruptured berry aneurysm is more common in females, patients with a history of coarctation of the aorta, and patients with polycystic kidney disease.

Diagnosis

- History and physical examination

- Evaluation by CT-scan or MRI confirms and localizes the lesion. An AVM may be seen, but aneurysms usually will not be identified. Diagnosis may be made with angiography and/or transcranial Doppler studies.

Treatment

- Because of the high risk of rebleeding from an aneurysm, surgical obliteration of the aneurysm is recommended.

- The short-term rebleeding risk of an unoperated aneurysm is approximately 40%, but after six months the risk is only 3% per year.

- Vasospasm is an important complication following subarachnoid hemorrhage and may result in secondary neurological deterioration.

- Cerebral perfusion is maintained by hemodilution, hypervolemia, elevation of blood pressure, and vasodilation with a calcium channel blocker.

Brain Abscess

General
- Brain abscess is a focal suppurative process within the brain parenchyma of varied etiology.
- This is generally a rare disease, though focal suppurative processes have emerged as an important type of infection in patients with AIDS.
- Pyogenic brain abscesses usually evolve over about a two-week period. The source of infection is identifiable in approximately 80% of cases.
- Causes include previous surgery, penetrating head trauma, extension from adjacent infections (otitis media, sinusitis, mastoiditis, and dental infection), valvular heart disease, arteriovenous malformation, hematogenous spread, and immune compromised states. The offending agent depends upon the source.

Clinical Manifestations
- Common symptoms of brain abscess include headache, fever, and focal neurological deficits; however, these symptoms are not consistently present.
- Patients may also present with altered mental status secondary to increased intracranial presure.

Diagnosis
- In evaluating a patient with symptoms such as these, both brain abscess and brain tumor must be considered.
- A history that would suggest a source of infection should be obtained and a thorough physical examination performed.
- A CT-scan or MRI is used to diagnose and localize the infection.

Treatment
- Surgery is the treatment for brain abscess in order to remove the purulent material, identify the organism, and reduce the mass effect.
- If the abscess is not easily accessible, CT-guided stereotaxic aspiration is the treatment of choice.
- Surgery is followed by antibiotic therapy targeted to the offending organism.

Disorders of the Spine

Disc Herniation

General
- The intervertebral disc is composed of the nucleus pulposus and the surrounding annulus fibrosus.
- Disc herniation occurs when the nucleus pulposus is extruded through a tear in the annulus fibrosus.

Clinical Manifestations
- Extrusion generally occurs posterolaterally and often compresses a nerve root, resulting in symptoms, usually pain.
- The pain occurs in the spine and often down one extremity and is exacerbated by straining and by movement of the affected part of the spine.
- Most symptomatic disc herniations occur in the lumbar spine, usually at the L4-5 and L5-S1 levels.
- In the case of lumbar herniation, the patient generally has low back and leg pain which is worse with weight bearing.
- The sciatic leg pain radiates down the posterior or lateral leg.
- The evaluation of low back pain begins by testing for point tenderness and evaluating range of motion.
- The examiner then attempts to raise the affected leg while the patient is lying down. If the patient experiences sciatic pain, lumbar disc herniation is likely.
- Pain in the affected leg when the unaffected leg is raised is pathognomonic for lumbar disc herniation.
- MRI and CT myelograms are most informative in evaluating lumbar disease.

Treatment
- Initial treatment is usually conservative and consists of several days of bed rest with activity as tolerated, analgesics, and anti-inflammatory agents.
- If there is no progress, if the condition worsens, or if there is marked weakness, surgery should be considered.
- The standard technique is discectomy by a posterior approach with removal of some of the adjacent lamina and removal of the disc herniation.

Tumors of the Nervous System

General

• Classification of Brain Tumors:

• Brain tumors that occur within the parenchyma of the brain are called intrinsic whereas those that occur outside of it are called extrinsic. Intrinsic tumors are usually more malignant and are more difficult to excise.

• Brain tumors can also be classified as infratentorial, those that occur in the posterior fossa and supratentorial, occurring above the tentorium cerebelli. Because of their location, infratentorial tumors are associated with increased ICP.

• In children, intrinsic tumors are most commonly infratentorial. These include:

  - Medulloblastoma

  - Cerebellar astrocytoma

  - Ependymoma

  - Brain stem glioma

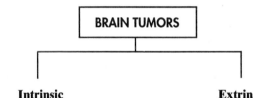

Intrinsic	**Extrinsic**
1. Metastasis	1. Meningioma
2. Glioblastoma multiforme	2. Pituitary adenoma
3. Oligodendroglioma	3. Acoustic Neuroma
4. Anaplastic astrocytoma	
5. Low grade astrocytoma	
6. Ependymoma	

Intrinsic Brain Tumors

Metastastaic Brain Tumors

✳• Metastatiac brain tumors are among the most common malignancies of the brain.

• Common primary tumors that metastasize to the brain include:
  - Melanoma
  - Thyroid
  - Lung
  - Breast
  - Gastrointestinal
  - Kidney

✳• The hallmark of metastatic brain tumors is the presence of multiple lesions on radiological studies.

Glioblastoma Multiforme (GBM)

✳• Glioblastoma multiforme is the most common and most aggressive type of brain tumor in adults.

• GBM is an undifferentiated tumor that grows very rapidly and has a high degree of recurrence.

• Patients diagnosed with GBM invariably die within 12 months of the diagnosis.

• GBM usually occurs in the fifth decade of life.

• Radiological studies reveal a ring enhancing lesion. However, these lesions are also commonly seen in brain abscesses or brain metastasis.

Oligodendroglioma

• Oligodendroglioma arises from the myelin-producing cells in the CNS, the oligodendrocytes.

✳• The hallmark of this type of tumors is the sudden onset of seizures in an adult without prior history of seizures.

Anaplastic astrocytoma

• A glioma is a tumor that arises from any of the glial cells that are found within the parenchyma of the brain. These include:
  - Astrocytes
  - Oligodendrocytes
  - Ependymal cells

• Anaplastic astrocytoma is also a highly aggressive tumor.

• Unlike GBM the 5-year survival rate of these tumors is about 18%.

• A benign form of a neoplasm arising from astrocyes is called **low grade astrocytoma** and occurs frequently in children.

Extrinsic Brain Tumors

Meningioma
- Meningioma is the most common extrinsic tumor. Following brain metastastasis, it is the second most common intracranial tumor in adults.
- Meningiomas commonly arise at the site of arachnoid granulations.
- These tumors are benign and completely resectable.
- Meningiomas are characterized for seizures due to the pressure that the tumor exerts in the cortex of the brain.
- There is a low rate of recurrence with these tumors. Most patients are disease free in 20 years after resection.

Pituitary Adenomas
- Most pituitary tumors are hormone-producing tumors and most are prolactinomas.
- The hallmark of these tumors is the clinical manifestations that result from the production of hormones (e.g., amenorrhea, galactorreha in females and impotence in men).
- Because of the close proximity of the pituitary gland to the optic chiasm, pituitary tumors may present with visual field problems.

Acoustic Neuromas
- Acoustic neuroma is a schwannoma of the vestibular nerve.
- The hallmark of acoustic neuroma is unilateral tinnitus with vertigo and hearing loss.

Clinical Manifestations
- The clinical manifestations are dependent on the type of brain tumor and some hallmark clinical manifestations are indicated above.
- Intrinsic tumors have the following general clinical manifestations:

Symptoms
- Headache
- Neurological deficits
- Changes in affect
- Decreased cognitive function
- Seizures

Signs
- Papilledema
- Increased ICP
- May present with hydrocephalus

Diagnosis

- History and physical examination
- CT-scans and MRI

Treatment

- The mainstay of treatment of brain tumors is surgery.
- Radiation therapy is recommended for some types of tumors such as metastatic brain tumors and GBM.

REFERENCES

1. Andreoli TE, et al., eds.: *Cecil Essentials of Medicine,* ed. 4. Philadelphia, W.B. Saunders Company, 1997.

2. Blackbourne LH: *Surgical Recall,* ed. 2. Baltimore, Williams & Wilkins, 1998.

3. Cohen JR: *Vascular Surgery for the House Officer,* ed. 3. Baltimore, Williams & Wilkins, 1997.

4. Cotran RS, et al., eds.: *Robbins Pathologic Basis of Disease,* ed. 6. Philadelphia, W.B. Saunders Company, 1998.

5. Doherty GM, et al.: *The Washington Manual of Surgery, ed. 2.* Philadelphia, Lippencott-Raven, 1999.

6. Fauci AS, et al., eds.: *Harrison's Principles of Internal Medicine,* ed. 14. New York, McGraw-Hill, 1998.

7. Fishman MC, et al: *Medicine,* ed. 4. Philadelphia, Lippincott-Raven Publishers, 1997.

8. Greenfield LJ, et al: *Review for Surgery: Scientific Principles and Practice.* Philadelphia, Lippincott-Raven Publishers, 1997.

9. Harken AH, Moore EE: *Abernathy's Surgical Secrets,* ed. 3. Philadelphia, Hanley & Belfus, 1996.

10. Heimer L. *The Human Brain and Spinal Cord.* New York, Springer-Verlag, 1983.

11. Jospe N, Forbes G: Fluids and Electrolytes—Clinical Aspects. *Pediatrics In Review* 17:395-402, 1996.

12. Lawrence PF: *Essentials of General Surgery,* ed. 2. Baltimore, Williams & Wilkins, 1992.

13. Lawrence PF: *Essentials of Surgical Specialties.* Baltimore, Williams & Wilkins, 1993.

14. Moore KL: *Clinically Oriented Anatomy,* ed. 3. Baltimore, Williams and Wilkins, 1992.

15. Myers AR: *NMS Medicine,* ed. 3. Baltimore, Williams & Wilkins, 1997.

16. O'Connell TX, et al.: *Classic Presentations and Rapid Review for the USMLE*

Step Alexandria, J&S Publishing, 1999.

17. Rose BD: *Clinical Physiology of Acid-Base and Electrolyte Disorders,* ed. 4. New York, McGraw Hill, 1994.

18. Sabiston DC Jr., Lyerly HK, eds.: *Textbook of Surgery: The Biological Basis of Modern Surgical Practice.* Philadelphia, W.B. Saunders Company, 1996.

19. Tanagho EA, McAninch JW. *Smith's General Surgery.* Norwalk, Appleton & Lange, 1995.

20. Tierney LM Jr., McPhee SJ, Papadakis MA: *Current Medical Diagnosis & Treatment 1996.* Stamford, Appleton & Lange, 1996.

21. Way LW, ed.: *Current Surgical Diagnosis & Treatment,* ed. 10. Norwalk, Appleton & Lange, 1994.

22. Wilcox RT, Traverso LW: Have the Evaluation and Treatment of Acute Appendicitis Changed with New Technology? *Surgical Clinics of North America* 77: 1355-1370, 1997.

23. Winawer SJ, et al.: *Colorectal Cancer Screening: Clinical Guidelines and Rationale.* Gastroenterology 112:594-692, 1997.

188

E-G

ECMO, 34
empyema, gallbladder, 99
endarterectomy, carotid, 117
enema, barium, 96
enterocolitis, necrotizing, 43
esophagitis, reflux, 64
esophagus, Barrett's, 64
euvolemia, 7
examination, neurological, 170
excess, volume, 14
exposure, 4
fibroadenoma, of breast, 131
fistula, in Crohn's disease, 90
, tracheoesophageal, 31
fluid, extracellular, 6
, intracellular, 6
foramen, of Bochdalek, 33
, of Morgagni, 33
fracture, skull, 173
gangrene, 119
gastroschisis, 40
Gleason, 144
glioblastoma multiforme, 182
grading, system of Gleason, 144
graft, coronary artery bypass, 113

H

Helicobacter pylori, 71
hematochezia, 86
hematoma, epidural, 171
, subdural, 172
hemorrhage, hypertensive intracerebral, 177
, subarachnoid, 178
hemorrhoids, 91
hemothorax, 2
hernia, congenital diaphragmatic, 33
, femoral, 60
, Grynfeltt's, 60
, hiatal, 62
, incarcerated, 60
, incisional, 60
, inguinal, direct, 45, 60
, indirect, 59

, Littré's, 61
, obturator, 61
, pantaloon, 60
, Petit's, 60
, Reichert's, 61
, Spigelian, 61
, stangulated, 60
, transtentorial, 169
herniatiation, intervertebral disc, 180
hydrocele, 46
hygroma, cystic, 158
hypercalcemia, 19
hyperkalemia, 18
hypermagnesemia, 21
hypernatremia, 17
hypertrophy, prostatic, 141
hypocalcemia, 20
hypokalemia, 17
hypomagnesemia, 22
hyponatremia, 16

I-L

ileus, 77
incontience, bladder, 149
index, ankle to brachial, 119
infarction, myocardial, 113
intussusception, 49
jaundice, 41, 100
lavage, diagnostic periotoneal (DPL), 5
ligaments, Cooper's, 129
lymphoma, 78

M-P

malformation, anorectal, 42
mammography, 133
mass, congenital neck, 30
mastectomy, 137
megacolon, toxic, 91
melena, 86
meningioma, 183
neuroma, acoustic, 183
obstipation, 76
obstruction, large bowel, 76
, small bowel, 76
oligodendroglioma, 182

Q-S

T-Z

J & S BOOKS NOW AVAILABLE FROM:

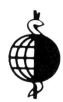 **FA Davis Company**:
1915 Arch Street, Philadelphia, PA 19103
www.FADavis.com, orders@fadavis.com
PH 1-800-323-3555, FX 1-215-440-3016).

- Also published by J & S Publishing Company, Inc., by the same authors, *CLASSIC PRESENTATIONS and RAPID REVIEW FOR THE USMLE, Step 2* (ISBN 1-888308-05-2, 1999, 215 pp, $ 25.00). Reviewers at www.amazon.com said:
  - **5 stars** "I used this book to study for the USMLE. I did not use any other study source and began studying only four days before the exam. This book was thorough but easy to get through, providing me with very valuable knowledge. The proof is in my results: I scored 228. If you want an easy way to get solid results, I suggest you get your hands on this book."
  - **5 stars** "Want to pass? Buy this book! The authors have really put their fingers on what you need to know to pass Step 2. They've focused on the high yield topics, with useful hints throughout, and organized it in an easy-to-read format."
  - **5 stars** "Excellent. I have read through this book while working on practice tests. I am convinced that reading this material is good for at least a 15 point improvement on the exam."
  - **5 stars** "Truly, a must have for any medical student. This book is an indispensable review for USMLE, Step 2, Step 3, and even just for the wards in general. The authors have boiled it down to what one really needs to know. The bullet format is very easy to read."

Other USMLE, Step 2 Books Available from J & S Publishing Company, Inc.

- *Surgery: Review for New National Boards*, Glenn W. Geelhoed, MD, FACS. ISBN 0-9632873-5-4, 246 pp., $ 25.00. This is clinically based collection of more than 500 questions and answers with many b&w illustrations and clinical vignettes. This book is an abridged version of *The Study of Surgery*.
- *The Study of Surgery*, Glenn W. Geelhoed, MD, FACS. ISBN 0-9632873-6-2. 392 pp., $ 40.00. This is a clinically based collection of more than 1000 questions and answers with many color and b&w illustrations and clinical vignettes.
- *Obstetrics and Gynecology: Review for New National Boards*, Ralph L. Kramer, MD, FACOG. ISBN 0-9632873-9-7, 190 pp., $ 25.00. This is a clinically based collection of more than 500 questions and answers with many b&w illustrations and clinical vignettes.

- These books are available at your local medical bookstore, from FA Davis Company (www.FADavis.com, e-mail orders@fadavis.com, PH 1-800-323-3555, FX 1-215-440-3016), from Internet booksellers, or direct from the publisher, J & S Publishing Company, Inc., 1300 Bishop Lane, Alexandria, VA 22302, PH 703-823-9833, FX 703-823-9834, e-mail jandspub@ix.netcom.com, www.jandspub.com. Credit card purchases are available from FA Davis or Internet booksellers.